T0146737

The Electrical Body
VS
Weightology

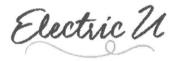

A JOURNEY II WHOLENESS

Electric U

Christine Maxwell

WESTBOW
PRESS®
A DIVISION OF THOMAS NELSON
& ZONDERVAN

This book is a work of non-fiction. Unless otherwise noted, the author
and the publisher make no explicit guarantees as to the accuracy of
the information contained in this book and in some cases, names
of people and places have been altered to protect their privacy.

Scripture taken from the King James Version of the Bible.

WestBow Press books may be ordered through
booksellers or by contacting:

WestBow Press
A Division of Thomas Nelson & Zondervan
1663 Liberty Drive
Bloomington, IN 47403
www.westbowpress.com
1 (866) 928-1240

Because of the dynamic nature of the Internet, any web addresses or
links contained in this book may have changed since publication and
may no longer be valid. The views expressed in this work are solely those
of the author and do not necessarily reflect the views of the publisher,
and the publisher hereby disclaims any responsibility for them.

Any people depicted in stock imagery provided by Thinkstock are models,
and such images are being used for illustrative purposes only.
Certain stock imagery © Thinkstock.

ISBN: 978-1-5127-9346-8 (sc)
ISBN: 978-1-5127-9345-1 (e)

Library of Congress Control Number: 2017910922

Print information available on the last page.

WestBow Press rev. date: 08/04/2017

In memory of Alfredo Bowman, born in Honduras in 1933, known by many as Dr. Sebi, a worldwide healer of many diseases for many people. I am thankful to him for imparting into my life the importance of understanding our bodies and on the matter of alkaline electrical foods. My life is changed forever because of your wisdom and knowledge. I will keep your legacy alive by sharing all the treasures I received from you with all whom God allows to come across my path. God used you to help me transition to an alkaline electrical lifestyle. Your seed is bringing forth a great harvest as the Word speaks, lest a seed fall to the ground and die there will be no harvest (John 12:24). I know I could have never done this on my own. I am forever grateful to God for using you to impart to me your wisdom and vast experience in the alkaline, electrical, and plant world. I will continue to search for the truth just as you did.

This book is my seed! I sow it for the greater harvest to come, for every life that will forever be changed as mine was.

Acknowledgments

First and foremost, God gets all the glory for truly inspiring and infusing me with His divine love that has forever transformed my life, and that love through me will help to transform others.

To Cedrick, my youngest son, and to Lorena, thank you for allowing God to use you to introduce me to the life of Dr. Sebi.

Words cannot express my gratitude, and love for Lisa, an incredible spiritual daughter, sister, and friend for believing and encouraging me. Also for her countless hours of hard work that she dedicated to seeing this book come to life.

To my friend and intercessor, Betty, I thank you for your prayers and the time you dedicated to helping me and encouraging me.

Introduction

Hello, beautiful butterflies, full of life's vibrant colors! Yes, you! You are beautiful, full of God's light and life. Yes, you! You are made in the image and likeness of God. I know life doesn't always make us feel beautiful. I agree that life can beat us down to the D place. You may be asking yourself, "What is the D place?" Let's name some of these places. Have you ever felt dead, down, discouraged, dismayed, disheartened, or damaged? Go ahead—name some of your D places. These are feelings we've all had at least once in our lives. The key is, what do we do with these feelings? Does anyone have an answer? There are answers, right? Do we tuck them away in our hearts, our stomachs, or maybe our heads? Let's us go through a door to discover where they are. God said, "Seek and you will find. Knock and the door will be open" (Matthew 7:7). You did not just happen to pick this book up. It was divine, and this is your divine appointment!

You asked for help and received this book. You were seeking when you received this book. Knocking is what you were doing when you came across this book. The door is open. Now the question is, will you walk through?

Most of us have asked for open doors before, but often we do not recognize the open doors. Doors come in many shapes and sizes in the natural world in which we live, and they can serve as a symbol of spiritual doors. Our life experiences speak to us and give us spiritual revelation, if we are open to have eyes to see, ears to hear, and a heart to comprehend. The earth is His and the fullness thereof. God uses everything in our lives to speak to us about us. On this journey, we will discover some of the doors that are open for you now. Some time ago, I was brought to a huge door. I looked in and saw through time all that was awaiting me. I was asked many times to walk through that door, but life's Ds were—well, I could say holding me back, but instead I will say I had not experienced enough of the Ds, so I would not walk through the door. Don't think for a moment that I was aware of it in the way that I am now. No, I was blinded. I could not see truth as truth. I met my divine appointment, and I will share what it looked like throughout this book. Be open, because divine appointments aren't always what we expect.

Have you ever felt like you were on a merry-go-round and just could not get off? I have been there, but I got off, and you can too! You may be saying, "You don't know my story." You are right, I don't; however, I do know we all are more alike than not. Life has cycles, and we all have experienced, at some point those cycles. Just like we can't stop winter, spring, summer, or fall from happening, we can't stop the cycles of life happening. We have been given power over these cycles, but most of us either don't know it or don't know how to use the power. Together we will embark on this new journey to discover ways to use this power given to us.

It's time to launch out into the deep, spread our wings, and soar! We no longer can, nor will, we allow fear to be the obstacle that hinders or stops us from becoming whole in our spirits, souls, and bodies. Are you ready to spread those beautiful wings and show the world your beauty? The world is waiting to see your unique colors. Divine timing awaits you! Selah!

My hope is this book will inspire you to see things in a new light. As I share my life-changing journey, it is my yearning that you will ascend that holy mountain to get what you need and build your temple (body) that you have been blessed with. This book is intended to help you make some life-changing decisions. If you make one change in your life for the good, then I am grateful to God for allowing this book to help you make that change.

CHAPTER 1

Inspiration

The Inner You
Being Inspired

It's time to dream bigger than ever before. Listen to the still, small voice that says, "This is the way walk in it." The doors are open, and we get to choose which door we will walk through! God told me to tell you the sky is the limit and it's time to take the limits and boundaries off. We are free spirit, soul, and body to soar. We have been created to soar; we have been made to soar. Our freedom was paid for over two thousand years ago. We are blessed and highly favored by the most-high God. What more do we need? If God is for us, who can be against us? Awaken the spirit of the entrepreneur! Love yourself enough to let nothing or no one stop you from dreaming and achieving what you dream. We can do it! Will it be a challenge? Yes, and even if it costs us all, we will be who God called and destined us to be. We are up for it! We no longer run from challenges; we run to them to overthrow and conquer all fears! If you see it as a challenge, that means you are dealing with fear, false evidence appearing real. How do we overcome what we fear? We must face it and walk through it or do it afraid! We can't quit.

What are you inspired to do? Think about the question for a moment. Don't say to prosper and be in good health—that's too broad. Be specific. Listen for a few more moments. Take some deep breaths, exhale, and be still for a few moments. Hear in the innermost part of yourself. God will speak. You may need to pause here, walk away, and allow the Spirit to speak to you. Waiting is something we have to exercise because the world is constantly moving faster, and most of us try to keep up. I don't know about you, but it has been a journey for me to learn the art of waiting. I have truly come to love that place. It is still and peaceful in that place. It may take some time, but if you wait on it, surely it will come. When you receive it, write it. It's important to revisit it daily and begin to speak it out of your mouth. Keep it before you. Maybe you are saying, "I tried that, and it didn't work." Why didn't it work? Could it be that you sabotaged it yourself? What I have discovered is writing it down builds you up in your most holy faith.

It takes time to build a house in this physical world, right? How long does it take? Most of us don't know how long it takes. Most people don't know how long it will take to change their situations. Well, in my profession I deal with builders, and depending on many factors, it could take four to six months, even a year, to build a home. We can liken our faith to building a house. There are many factors involved. The time frame can vary depending on those factors. What are some of your factors? Ask yourself what obstacles you need to overcome. List them—we'll wait. Now, what will it take to remove those obstacles one at a time? This is how you will build your faith. Say, "I have overcome these," and name them. It is important to be willing to change your perspective. Today they are no longer obstacles. Remember: building your house takes time. Giving up is not an option. We are often ensnared by our own words. I used to say all the time, "I don't want to own houses. It's too much work."

I would say this to myself year after year until I heard this small voice say, "Is it too hard?" The Spirit said in a soft voice, "When you sell a house, you tell people all the time to persevere, that anything worth having is worth fighting for. But the real reason you do not want to own any more houses is because of the challenges they present, or so you made yourself believe."

I pondered the words spoken to me for days, weeks, perhaps even months! One day it sank into my spirit to change my perspective. I began to declare and speak these words: "I *will* face every obstacle with a new mind-set. I will overcome them, and I will get the victory. I will own properties all over this world one at a time. Just like He told Joshua: 'Every place that the sole of your foot shall tread upon, that have I given unto you, as I said unto Moses'" (Joshua 1:3).

Here is another inspirational key. We must shift our thinking from faith in God to the faith of God. Wait, what? Let me explain: faith in God means you believe God to do it. Faith of God means you speak as God speaks by doing it. Jesus said He didn't do anything unless He saw His Father do it. Jesus did it; He did not believe God was going to do it. His faith was not *in* God doing; He had the faith *of* God—He did it. The scriptures tell us that God did not let one of Samuel's words fall to the ground. Why? Because Samuel had the faith of God, He did it! He was speaking as God, not believing in God or waiting for God to do it. Samuel spoke, and it was done (1 Samuel 3:19). God and heaven backed what seemingly were Samuel's words. However, they were not Samuel's words but rather God's words. It was God speaking through Samuel. This is the faith of God! No longer will I have the faith *in* God to get it done; I have the faith *of* God. It's done! This house is being built one brick at a time from the inside out. Selah.

We all have been given gifts and talents to use in the earth. What are your gifts? Are you using them? I believe the purpose God has sent us to the earth for is linked to our gifts and talents. I thank God for the gifts that have been given to me. I name them and thank God for blessing me to know them and walk in them daily. I often meet people who do not have a clue who they are or why they are here. Many don't believe they have any gifts. Do you know your purpose and gifts? If you know, do you take it for granted? Are you fulfilling your purpose? I believe the word of God is clear regarding this matter. I believe it is God's desire for us to know our destiny and to live life to fulfill that purpose. God's plan for us is clearly stated in the word: "I know the plans I have for you, declares the Lord, plans to prosper you and not to harm you, plans to give you hope and a future" (Jeremiah 29:11).

My purpose is tied to my gift to sell and buy real estate, which I have been blessed to do for over thirty years. It took me a very long time to understand how my purpose was tied to this experience. Real estate deals with land, and God uses land to speak to us about who we are. We are the land. It has been stolen from us, and we must get it back! I wrote a book called *A Journey through Joshua*, which showed me how Joshua was not just a book to read but a life to live. We are the land God talks about in the book of Joshua! It's our experience told in a metaphor using land. How is God speaking to you daily about your purpose and using your gifts and talents? Ask God, and I know you will be shown. Our life experiences will tell us daily who we are and what God is saying to us. Listen carefully! Don't take anything for granted. Our children, our jobs, our bodies, and so on all speak to us daily. Are you listening? Do you understand what life is saying to you? Be inspired, stay inspired, and let your life's purpose be an inspiration.

Reflect

_____

_____

_____

_____

_____

_____

_____

_____

_____

_____

_____

_____

_____

_____

CHAPTER 2

A Step onto a New Path

I have embarked upon a new journey. Walking on this new path is one of the biggest steps I have ever taken. This journey is one to become whole in my body, soul, and spirit, which has and will enable me to do more than ever before. This is an invitation for you to join me on this journey. Remember: it is by divine appointment you have received this book. So it is your time! I promise you will have no regrets! Will you face obstacles? Yes, you will. However, the rewards outweigh all challenges you will face. Your body, soul, and spirit will all scream, "Thank you!"

Let's journey back as far as we can and look at some important truths that will help us on this journey. Adam and Eve walked in the cool of the day with God. Have you ever asked yourself how they did this? It is my belief that through spiritual revelations their vibrations allowed them to walk in multiple dimensions. We know Haggai 1:8 talks about ascending a holy mountain and bringing down timber to build God's temple. What is this verse telling us? These are levels or vibrations that enable us to ascend and descend in the spirit realm. Remember: we are spirit, soul, and body. If they did it, it is my understanding we can too! The word of God tells us, "No good thing will the Father withhold from us." A journey to a higher vibration or frequency is our ultimate purpose to walk with God daily. Our Creator made us in His image and likeness for a purpose. I believe that purpose is to enable us to walk in the cool of the day with them, Father, Son, and Spirit. The cool of the day to me represents perfect harmony, oneness, and total unity. It is a place where there is nothing missing. If we think about a beautiful, cool, sunny day in the earth in which we live, what comes to mind? I picture peace, joy, and total fulfillment in every area of my life. Most of us were taught Eve was deceived when she ate the forbidden fruit. I see it as they ate what was appealing to their natural eyes, and it has caused most if not all of us to do likewise. We are diverted by what looks good, tastes good, feels good, etc. We eat with our five senses in full gear. But is this the right way? Have we been hoodwinked by what the world says looks, tastes, feels, and sounds real?

As a student who was open to learn, I discovered some interesting truths that I will be sharing with you on our journey to wholeness and debunking a few myths along the way. One of the biggest myths in our lives is what I have named weightology. We will talk more about this later. It is one myth we have all fallen for at some point in our lives. Our bodies are perfect machines that have been entrusted to us. The myth is "I am too fat or too skinny."

Our pursuit to lose weight often consumes many of us at some point in our lives. We have bought expensive weight-loss drugs, gaining perhaps some degree of success, only to gain more than we started with. We never stopped to realize that this is a cycle and we have been given the power to overcome it. One important lesson we must learn is weight is not the problem; it is a symptom of something far greater. No matter how much money you spend to get that perfect body, until you understand the deeper root, you will find yourself back where you started.

The root I have discovered is in what we are eating. We have adapted to the concept of eating what is appealing to our senses. We must spend some time examining what the world system calls "good." For example, many of us have a starch-based diet. We may have grown up eating a starch, vegetable, and meat, which we thought was good. Well, let's take on the student position and open our minds to learning some new and perhaps challenging truths. Let's start by asking the question, what is starch, and how does the body assimilate or absorb it? Most of us have been told it turns into sugar, right? Let's understand what starch and sugar are and how the body responds to them. I know I am stepping on some sacred cows now. Starch and sugar are what we all love. However, do we understand why we love it? Well if we truly want to go on this journey to wholeness, then we should look at these two creatures closely. We are always students first, and when we learn, we are compelled to teach. Here are a few interesting facts.

Did You Know Food Has a Vibration?

Starch is made up of long chains of glucose, which is a simple sugar. It's used to produce many of the sugars in processed foods. Dissolving starch in warm water gives wheat paste, which can be used as a thickening, stiffening, or gluing agent. It's also used as an adhesive in the papermaking process

Could this be the core of why we are gaining weight? I chose the word *weightology* for the title of the book because to me it represents something made up to describe what we have been trying so desperately to get rid of, weight, which is a by-product of man-made inventions.

Stay tuned for more interesting facts about these two creatures.

> *Study to show thyself* approved unto God, a
> workman that needed not to be ashamed,
> rightly dividing the word of truth.
> —2 Timothy 2:15

Healthier Choices to Replace Starch

Spelt, kamut, teff, and amaranth are all ancient grains that have been around a lot longer than starch. They are now being ground into flour to give us a healthier choice. Each of these grains is much easier for the body to assimilate, or absorb. They will not make you gain weight. However, they should be used in moderation as you transition to a plant-based diet.

I have used a variety of spelt, kamut, and chickpea/garbanzo bean flour and flakes and found they work well in recipes that call for things like white flour, which is a starch. Give them a try to see which ones you might like.

I could not tell the difference in the taste.

Wikipedia Definitions

Spelt is a type of wheat that has been cultivated since 5000 BC. It's ancient—meaning it is very old. It has six sets of chromosomes. Spelt has a more soluble protein matrix.

Kamut is an ancient grain type; this grain is twice the size of modern-day wheat and is known for its rich nutty flavor. In order to sell a grain under the trademark Kamut, it must fulfil several conditions: It must belong to the ancient Khorasan variety of wheat (i.e., no breeding, no genetic manipulation). It must only be grown as a certified organic grain. It must contain a protein range of 12 to 18 percent. It must be 99 percent free of modern wheat's contaminating varieties. It must be 98 percent free of all signs of disease.

The most popular ancient grains used today include spelt, Khorasan wheat (Kamut), millet, barley, and teff. They are a healthier choice for us to use instead of food made with starch.

Chickpeas are a nutrient-dense food, providing rich content (20 percent or higher of the Daily Value, DV) of protein, dietary fiber, folate, and certain dietary minerals, such as iron and phosphorus. Thiamin, vitamin B6, magnesium, and zinc contents are moderate.

Garbanzo bean flour or besan is pulse flour made from ground chickpeas

Reflect

_____

_____

_____

_____

_____

_____

_____

_____

_____

_____

_____

_____

_____

Electric U

CHAPTER 3

No More Diets!

I have discovered some amazing things about this electrical machine the world calls the body. It is truly so much more than a body. It is best described as an electrical machine because it is powerful! I have, at best, only scratched the surface of what He has allowed me to understand about it. This electrical machine speaks to us; however, most often we are not listening. Did you know our bodies are created to heal themselves? Because of what we have accepted as truth, our bodies are now sick and filled with diseases and infirmities that have caused them to malfunction from their original purpose. But it's not too late—we can regain all! This includes the original way our bodies were created to function. Let's fight to get our original bodies back! Anything worth having is worth fighting for, right? It will be a battle and perhaps a war for some, but one worth fighting. I promise all of heaven's armies will fight for you. I am living proof of what God has and is doing, in the spirit, soul, and body. I truly have been given eyes to see and ears to hear and a heart that truly understands much more than ever before about our Creator God's creation He calls *man*. We must truly be born again, from flesh to spirit. We can't wage war against a system that has been in place since creation in our flesh, our natural man (soul equals mind, will, and emotions). Therefore, it is important that we fight the good fight of faith and not turn back but press toward the mark of the higher calling, which is what Christ came to show us, dying to our mind, will, and emotion to live His way. It is not accomplished overnight, so don't think, *I can't. It's too hard!* Perhaps you have tried more times than you can count to lose weight, to walk in your purpose, or to get out of debt, just to name a few. We have all been there, at the place of giving up, the D place! We have more help than ever before, or should I say, we now are being awakened to know that all of heaven and the cloud of witnesses are helping us. We stand on their shoulders to do more than we could do before. Truly, greater is He that is in you than he that is in the world. We know we wrestle not against flesh and blood but against principalities and powers, rulers of the darkness of this age, but now we know that we don't fight alone. Ask God to show you the mighty ones like He showed the servant that was with Elisha in 2 Kings 6:17. We must understand what we are fighting against and how to fight.

We have been given an electrical body, and it requires electrical food. You may ask, "What is electrical food?" The door is open. Now is the time to walk through, to discover a whole new world waiting for us.

Electrical Food + Electric Body = Higher Vibration

Did you know Creator God created us in His image and likeness? He is the Spirit, which is energy, and energy is electrical and vibrates at a high frequency. Our spirit is made in His image and likeness.

In the Bible, in Genesis 1:29 it says He provided us with every herb bearing seed that contains all the nutrients the body needs. The seed is electrical, the seed is energy, and it is full of life, for every cell and organ in our bodies. He said, "I have given you every herb bearing seed, which is upon the face of all the earth, and every tree, in which is the fruit of a tree yielding seed …" In Revelation 22:2, He said, "The leaves are for the healing of the nations." He knew our struggle would be foods that would appeal to our five senses.

The seed, which is electrical, is the solution. It has the ability to reproduce and multiply all we would ever need. What was introduced to Eve in the Bible was a counterfeit. Eve chose based on her five senses, which were passed down to us. The counterfeit causes us to live by our five senses, which dictate what is good for us. It is not so easy to recognize what is good, because when we accept the counterfeit, it blinds us to the truth of what God created for us. Now we are being awakened to the truth. Remember, I told you our help is here, or should I say we are beginning to know our help. I believe once you receive this knowledge, it will provoke you to accept the truth. However, the natural man that has been conditioned by this world will scream, "I can't," but if I did it, anyone can do it. Perhaps, if "I can't," is sounding too loud for you to ignore, then you may have to be given another pill or two from a physician before you discover you can and you must. The truth will set you free, and the truth is, the counterfeit foods that look, taste, and smell good are killing us, making us sick, and causing us to be blinded to the truth. We need to eat foods He created for us, plant-based foods that are highly electrical, meaning they are alkaline, above seven on the pH scale, which will allow the body to easily assimilate them. God gave us seed and put seed in the earth, but He never said anything about how the seed would look, taste, or smell. But now, we choose by our senses to determine what is good and what we will or will not eat. Understand this truth—the more we consume foods that are created by God, the more our eyes will be opened to the truth given to us in the beginning, and the more our bodies will come alive. Most of our bodies are in survival mode. The body has elasticity; however, we don't know how long before the elastic will break. Breaking could be sickness, disease, or even death.

On my journey to wholeness, I have discovered some electrical foods, and I have tested them myself, eating most for months to see how my body would respond. What I discovered was astonishing. Not only did my body feel better, but I lost weight without trying. Surprising to me, I went from a size ten to a size five within months without trying. I was not focused on losing weight. I wanted to feel better; I wanted the pain to leave my body. Like most, my family history was quite long. I realized the deficiencies in my body came down the pipeline and had a seat at the table in my life because of my choices. I did not know I opened the door. Many of you have opened the door also. You may have convinced yourself otherwise by saying, "Well, my mother, who is now deceased, had it, and my father, who is deceased, had it, so it is inevitable for me to have the same things or worse. It's in my genes." Let's just say that to some degree that is true. Most of what we believe is genetic stems from what was passed down from generation to generation, their way of life, which became our way of life, and what they got we now get. If my father had diabetes and my mother had rheumatoid arthritis, is it guaranteed I will get it? That is what they tell us most likely will happen. What I know to be truth now is that if I follow the path/lifestyle they followed that was handed down to them from their parents, it is pretty guaranteed I will get what they had.

Remember the cycles I talked about earlier? Well, here is a cycle. If I don't understand that I must do something totally different than my parents did, it is a guarantee that I will be sitting in their seat. My body is weak because they were sick when my mother conceived me. This is a strike against me coming into this natural body.

If I continue their lifestyle, chances are I won't make it to their age, because sickness and disease are awaiting me. That elastic is getting weaker through every generation. This is a cycle that must be broken. This is a huge crisis. The body can only last so long on its current path. There are also other factors that are breaking down that elastic. We will visit some of those later. If we can't see the patterns, we are headed for a road of sickness and disease, if we are not already there. It is very important to understand what we are dealing with. It is not our fault, and it is not our forefathers' fault. Don't look for someone to blame; look for a solution that will change the course of life. You are the solution! You can change the course of life.

For me, it was important to understand what, why, and how. I found that when the body assimilates the foods that are alkaline and highly electrical, it begins to heal itself and slowly rids itself of all the toxins and diseases that the nonelectrical food caused in the body. This fascinating machine that has been given to us is amazing beyond belief. Interested in continuing this journey with me? Want to know more about our fascinating electrical machine?

This is a good place to pause and think about some of the knowledge you have gained up to this point. Write it down so you can keep it in front of you. Selah.

Reflect

_____

_____

_____

_____

_____

_____

_____

_____

_____

_____

_____

_____

CHAPTER 4

Weightology

Weightology—something that has been coined that is not real, just like weight! Yes, I said made-up, and yes, I said it's not real. I can hear some of you saying, "What do you mean?" When I looked in the mirror, I saw lots of weight that I wished was not real. What I know now as truth is that weight is not real, and you will understand my conclusion soon.

I discovered wholeness was far more important than weight to me. Don't get me wrong—I knew I needed to lose some weight, but it was not my focus. I, like most of you, loved food, so giving up what I loved was at the bottom of my agenda. When I started this journey, I didn't tell anyone my plan, because I honestly did not think I could achieve wholeness, but I was wrong! Now it's, "Hello, my *new* fabulous life!" I am feeling great and looking great!

It's all about your perspective. Shift your perspective from what you can't change, and just focus on becoming whole, which is our promise from our Creator, and the bonus will be weight loss without trying.

Eating to live instead of living to eat will bring you to a place called wholeness.

It's time to give up the game you have been playing involving losing weight. Don't spend another dollar on a pill that will "guarantee" weight loss. We are creators, and we are creating a new game called becoming whole, and the bonus points will be weight loss. Know this: the Heavenly Host and the cloud of witnesses are cheering you on! It's time to get a new attitude. It's time to design a new strategy for your new game. This game must be invented by you. You get to write the rules and strategy to ensure victory. Let's gather our team players, and let's make up the rules to the game. Without a doubt, if we are making up the rules, we will win without trying. Who makes up the rules to lose? *No one*! We don't have to struggle because we have developed the rules.

Life through the world's eyes is a game, and the creators of the world's game sat down and created a strategy that would ensure their victory! They made it seem like we could win their game and at times in our lives we fell for it, but we did not win many victories at all. Many games are developed to look easy and mislead you into thinking you can win while all along they have written it to ensure their victory and gain only. In the beginning, it *looked* achievable, but after a lifetime of trying, you wake up one day and realize something is wrong with the game you are playing. No matter how hard you play some games, the end has been determined by those who created the game. No one creates something to be defeated.

Creator God created us and has bestowed upon us the ability to be creators of our own path and our own destiny. The Bible was a guide that was given to us to show us just how to create our destiny. Now it's time to stop allowing others to write the rules of *our game/life*. We have been made the greatest creators through countless defeats; we have forgotten or have been made to think we are not competent enough to win. Then we begin to have self-doubt and allow the world system to create our game, and because of that, we have been defeated in most if not all areas of our life. The world system's games of life are called good health, better finances, best education, etc. Well, it's our time to take to the courts and create a new game written by us, and the end of the game is sweet victory. Let's look at what the world system did. They developed a strategy that would look achievable, but hidden behind the scenes were hidden strategies that would cause defeat for some but victory for those who created the game. Get your pen or pencil and begin creating. Let me remind you, He said, "Everything you name, that is what it will be" (Genesis 2:20). Adam was taught how to develop the rules of his life. Whatever he called a thing, the Master, Creator of heaven and earth, backed him up by saying, "Let it be!" Remember, He said in Genesis 1:3, "Let there be light and the light was." He has told us to name the game and the rules and how it will be played and He will back us up. Then He told Adam to cultivate (tend to it, don't allow anyone to come in and change the game or take it from you). They have rewritten our game for their gain. They presented it to us in a beautiful array of colors by making it appealing to the eye. It looks beautiful and easy, and once we bite (accept) it as our game, we go on a new journey of playing by the rules that have been created by others, only to one day wake up and realize, "I can't win this game." We want out of their game, but we don't know how to stop playing, because it looks good and everyone is playing it, so we have to keep playing, hoping God will cause us to win one day. We must realize and understand it was written for their gain, not ours.

How do we create a new game, one may ask? Well given the conditioning of our mind, it will be arduous. However, we are now up for the challenge. First make up in your mind that you will no longer play their game, no matter how good it looks. I tell my grands all the time that everything that looks good and tastes good is not always good for you. First, we shift our perception of the game. We don't look at it through the eyes of defeat, which is the way we have been for so long. We have been conditioned to look through fearful eyes in every area of our lives. We now have been awakened, and now we can rewrite the games of our lives one play at a time.

Let's look at the system in place in the medical field. This is a big one! Prepare to open your mind to what I will share now. Pause for a moment, and take a deep breath. This may be a hard pill to swallow, but you have swallowed many I am sure, so this won't be any harder than the others.

Think about this. You go to the doctor for one thing and come out with a pill that potentially can create a list of others. Somehow, in our conditional thinking, we justify this by telling ourselves, "Well, I will take a chance and pray God doesn't allow me to get any of these other things listed on the prescription." Question, if God allowed you to have the thing you went to the doctor for in the first place, how can you believe He won't allow you to get the others? Ask yourself, does that really make sense?

God did not give you any sickness or disease. Sickness and disease can often be traced back to the decisions and the choices we have made in conjunction with our senses that have been outplayed by the world's system. Until we wake up to realize we have been created to create our world, we will keep playing the game they created for their gain, not ours! Ouch, that hurt! The truth doesn't always initially feel good, but it will produce a good result if we are willing to accept it and receive it. Where do we begin? Again, change your perspective of the game. Create the strategy for the new game, "whole ball."

The new game plan is to eat to live and no longer live to eat! Everyone who plays the game by this principle is assured victory. How do I eat to live? We must go back to what we understand is the beginning. This is where the Creator created us and gave us the strategy to create our game. He showed us how to live life to the fullest. I will reiterate it again: we have to develop our own strategies. We are tricked when we follow our senses. How it looks and how it smells always get us in trouble. Remember, the game is now called, "Whole ball, our journey to wholeness, body, soul, mind, and spirit." We are on our way to discovering true treasures. Selah.

Reflect

_____

_____

_____

_____

_____

_____

_____

_____

_____

_____

_____

_____

_____

_____

Electric U

CHAPTER 5

Creating the Strategy for Your Game

Let's again look at the strategy they used in the beginning of time and examine it closely because in it is a true buried treasure that we can unearth. In Genesis 1:11, Creator God created the earth to bring forth everything we would need—herbs with seed, fruit-bearing trees with seed. Everything was given to us (every seed-bearing herb). Here lies a strategy for our "whole ball" game. Continuing in verse 29, He gave man every green herb, and seed to bring forth fruit for food. As we look at the truth of what food is believed to be, one must conclude we have gone astray from the original plan for us. Could this be why most, if not all of us are sick in our bodies? Have we been given something other than what the seeds produce and over time it has caused multiple symptoms in our bodies? Could this be the reason we find ourselves sitting in front of a doctor, hoping he or she can diagnose us?

The truth is, doctors did not create a body, but the world system says they have a license to diagnose the body. Remember, they wrote the rules to their game for their gain. What was the motive that was hidden from us? Was it because they cared so much for us and wanted to help us put them out of a job? No, that is what we so wanted to believe, so we fell for it in desperation. Who creates a game to lose? No one. If they have the capability or wanted to heal you, they would be out of a job. The game was not written with that in mind. The game was written for their financial gain. It's a system created for only certain ones to gain. I want to be clear and say this does not mean doctors are all bad, but I am saying once they get caught up in this broken system, their hands can easily be tied. Jesus said, "It took Me taking stripes on My body (horrific pain) for you to have access to your healing." Think about that truth. He showed us how they would cause our bodies to be in tremendous pain.

Wow! Pause and think about this.

If we meditate about it deeply, if everyone was healed by doctors, what would the doctors do? The true motive was hidden from us. We fell for it because we could not see, we were desperate and afraid, we wanted to be healed, and we did not want the pain anymore. Many of us have gone from doctor to doctor to doctor, only to find they do not have the power to heal. They put a bandage on the problem so we could not see or feel for a while, which caused us not to see truth, which is what their game was created to do. When the bandage is removed, you can see what is there and has been there all along. It was masked to prevent us from seeing what was brewing under the surface. Can you see why it is necessary to create our own game? It is time to create our own game in every area of our lives.

The other areas we need to address, like education, finances, business, and religion, all have rules for their gain, not ours. Thus, one game at a time, with God's help, we will open our eyes and develop a strategy for our new game, "whole ball." This one we will prosper and be in good health. I must advise you, it will take dying to what you are accustomed to doing. You have to create a new normal. It won't be easy, but it is achievable because the greater one is living in us and the host of heaven is with us, causing us to be able to do all things through *Him*. Stand firm with your mind focused. You don't want to play their games anymore. It won't be effortless because you have played it all your life and all around you, it is being played, but once your vibrations rise, you will see that you have all the help you need to not only create your game but help others' eyes to be open to the truth. When you learn, you have a responsibility to teach. The proof will be your new fabulous life of wholeness (the condition of being sound in body. The quality or state of being without restriction, exception, or qualification (*Merriam-Webster Dictionary*). To summarize this, wholeness is nothing missing and everything complete as God created you. Write a few strategies down to your game. Write some rules of how you will play your game. It may take you sitting still and pondering for a while, but this is a sacrifice you won't regret. Your willpower to stay focused, to receive the strategies for your game, will be your first victory.

It's time to regain our momentum now that we know the Master Creator created us and provided us with the necessary tools to succeed in this world. Jesus was the greatest example of how to create, and the Holy Spirit will be our Helper. He said, "The Kingdom of God is nigh unto you" (Luke 21:31). He is the King of the kings, so He will lead us. In Philippians 4:16 it says, "Be anxious for nothing, but in all things through prayer and thanksgiving let your request be made known."

The whole ball game is a game for everyone to play to win. Remember, the strategy is, "Eat to live, not live to eat" any longer. This will cause you to vibrate at a higher frequency, gaining points against your opponent, and will keep you from playing their game, "live to eat." You can't see with your physical eyes, but you will be vibrating at a higher frequency than before. Your evidence will be more energy, weight loss, clearer thoughts, and a lot more dreams and visions. Jesus said, "I don't do anything unless I see my Father do it." Well, if you are asking yourself, "How could He see His Father and what He was doing?" I would say it was the frequency that He was vibrating at that gave Him the ability to see!

Vibrating at a higher frequency allows you to ascend to higher realms. Christ lived in two realms, the spirit and the flesh/earth. You may say, "I am not worthy." Well, again, those kinds of thoughts come out of the conditioning of your mind all your life! You have been eating unhealthy foods of untruths that have fed your soul and body, not allowing your spirit to soar and live/walk in the cool of the day with the One that created you.

God, break every condition, every chain off our minds, and cause us to know and believe and live in the freedom You gave us to walk in the cool of the day with You as we did in the beginning.

Now receive and believe you can, and you will. We no longer permit doubts and fears to rob us of who we are. If God told Adam to create it, He told us to create it. You are fearfully and wonderfully made in His image and His likeness! He did not make you like Him to think and accept what and who the world system's game says you are! Every time that kind of thought of defeat and skepticism arises, and it will daily (we wrestle not against flesh and blood, Ephesians 6:12), you must replace each flesh thought with a God thought. For example, the two infamous words I hear all the time from people are, "I can't." I ask who told you those words, and why can't you? God said you can do all things through Him (Philippians 4:13), right? Why do you choose to believe you can't over you can? It's a choice. I can hear some of you saying, "Circumstances are real." Well again I say, who told you that? I believe I must call those things that be not as though they were (Romans 4:17), which means circumstances can and do change daily! Are circumstances what you have created through what you have believed and spoken into existence? Hmm ... something for you to think about.

Remember what I said earlier, what I spoke most often, "I don't want any more properties …"? And guess what? I got what I spoke. I did not get anymore, but now I speak, "I will get properties all over this world," and I will! Remember, He created us to create our world. What you have eaten has created who you are, both the natural foods you put in your mouth and foods/words you have eaten that have created your world. Did it take you a short time to create the world you live in now? If not, know that it will take time for you to undo, unlearn, and create your new world through the game called whole ball. *We* have again been conditioned to believe we can have it our way suddenly and quickly. McDonald's and Burger King have given us a false sense of how life is played. Playing with the world system rules won't work for our gain. Commit to the journey for however long it takes to create your game strategy so that you win in the end. Be specific. Write the details of the game you are creating. It is so important to write it and keep it in front of you and speak it daily.

> Write the vision make it plain
> on tablets though it tarry wait
> for it for it shall surely come.
> —Habakkuk 2:2

> So, a man thinketh so is he.
> —Proverbs 23:7

We have another generation coming behind us that needs to know the how, what, and when of our lives to help them to climb on our shoulders and our ancestors' shoulders, to create more than we will. Let me give you some facts from scientists and others that may help you on your journey.

Everything that exists in the physical, mental, emotional, and spiritual realms does so also on a vibratory basis. It is obvious if you consider that electrons are always moving and vibrating according to biowaves.com. Albert Einstein said everything is energy. Remember his formula $E=mc^2$? He believed that energy and matter were interchangeable. Everything is vibrating energy, including our bodies. Every word and every thought carries a certain vibrational frequency.

A Japanese scientist named Dr. Masaru Emoto proved this when he did an experiment with water. He found out that water is affected by words. He took water droplets and exposed them to various words. He froze them for three hours and then examined the crystal formations under a microscope. The results were totally astounding. When positive words were spoken over the water, it formed beautiful patterns. Negative words produced ugly patterns. Since our bodies are approximately 70 percent water, we know that our bodies are greatly affected by negative speech. He did another experiment with rice where he spoke "I love you" to a jar of rice for thirty days. To another jar of rice, he spoke the words "You fool." After thirty days, the rice in the "I love you" jar was white and the rice in the "You fool" jar was black and rotten. (Facts taken from Dr. Emoto's book *The Hidden Messages in Water*.)

It can be scientifically documented that everything has either positive or negative frequencies. Foods even have frequencies. Fresh food has a higher frequency than processed foods. On the other hand, coffee has a negative frequency. Prayer raises a person's frequency by 15 MHzs according to Dr. David Stewart. If our frequency gets low, we get sick. A healthy body has a frequency between 62 to 68 MHz. If a person's frequency dips to 58 MHz, cold symptoms develop. Flu symptoms appear at 57 MHz, and cancer may enter the body when the frequency falls below 42 MHz. The process of dying begins at 25 MHz and goes to zero at death. (Taken from Dr. David Stewart's book *Healing Oils of the Bible*.)

> God speaks to you at the speed of
> thought. Thought moves at the
> speed of light. As quickly as light
> illuminates a room, a single thought
> can illuminate your life. You are
> always only one thought away from
> living the life of your dreams—one
> decision away from destiny.
> — Dr. Cindy Trimm

James Allen wrote in his timeless classic, *As a Man Thinketh*, "All that a man achieves or fails to achieve is a direct result of his own thoughts. Your life moves in the direction of your thoughts. Thoughts are the ever-present currents that move you either closer or further away from your best future. Your life is what your thoughts make it." James Allen also observed that a person "will find that as he alters his thoughts toward things and other people, things and other people will alter towards him." This is the basic premise of the law of attraction. This phenomenon is rooted in the findings of quantum physics—which found that nothing in the universe is static since all matter is vibrating energy—raw energy that responds to the vibrations of our thoughts, so that consequently "what we now see did not come from anything that can be seen" (Hebrews 11:3 NLT). It is the essence of faith, "the substance of things hoped for, the evidence of things not seen" (Hebrews 11:1 NKJV).

Now, do you believe enough to create your wholelistic life? Write the rules to your whole ball game now! Try it for thirty days! What do you have to lose? Many of us are overweight and sick in our bodies, and our souls, minds, will, and emotions. It can't hurt any more than we have already hurt ourselves with help from the systems in place in this world. Remember, their game is written for their gain, not ours.

Reflect

_____

_____

_____

_____

_____

_____

_____

_____

_____

_____

_____

_____

_____

_____

Electric U

CHAPTER 6

Wholelistic life

Goal: Uproot the hell of the past! Uprooting everything that was passed down to us through generations is our goal. Now that we know better, we have to do better. I don't know about your view of disease and sickness, but my view is sickness and disease is hell. It is a place of suffering and torment daily. The definition of hell in *Webster's Dictionary* is "a place or state of misery, torment, or wickedness." I will say it again—we must uproot the hell of the past!

One may say, "How do I get started?" First, let go of all expectations and take one step at a time. If you have any other expectations, except a wholelistic life, you will set yourself up for failure. Let's set a few more guidelines to this game. Let's try some new things for thirty days. Open your heart to receive what your flesh will reject. When your natural mind says, "No way," stop and sit there for a minute. Ask yourself, "Why do I think I can't?" Now, choose not to accept the, "No way." Let it go. Say to yourself, "I can and I will receive this new step I have taken." Now take a few slow, deep breaths and exhale slowly. Okay, now let's open our hearts to receive the first step toward uprooting the hell of the past and receiving this life of wholeness.

First rule: remove some unhealthy foods out of your life for the next thirty days. This may seem too difficult for some; however, try before you say the words, "I can't."

Let go of all starches … ouch! You can and will do it for thirty days. Go back and read the definition of starch! That may help give you the ability to go on this thirty-day journey. I promise, you will be amazed by the results that come out of this leg of the journey. You won't just feel better, but you will notice a change in your physical body as well because you will not be storing any excess sugar. I will share some suggestions that may help you as you transition.

Second rule—replace the starches with high-energy, electrical foods, like kale, collards, and callaloo. Any of the dark-leaf veggies will be a tremendous benefit to your cells. It will even be good to juice and make smoothies with them. The darker the leaf, the more nutrients, and the higher energy it carries to the body's cells. The body will thrive and wake up and begin to function the way it was created to function. Everyone who has tried it for thirty days has said how much better they feel after four consistent weeks. Appreciate all kinds of salads. However, exclude iceberg lettuce. It has no nutrients and causes bloating. One vegetable I have come to love is spaghetti squash, when it is in season. All squash are great electrical foods. Eat things that are not necessarily appealing to the taste buds at first but are good for the body. Your taste buds will conform, I promise. Step out of your comfort zone and try veggies you have never tried before and fruits too! Do some research on your own of veggies that are high in nutrients, especially in the area you know your body is deficient. We all need calcium and iron, but let's get them from all-natural sources. Eat as much and as often as you like of the high-energy electrical foods. They are feeding your cells. Remember, you are eating to live now. The body will slowly start to wake up and begin functioning the way it was created to.

I have learned if we replace the junk we have become accustomed to eating, like the starches and sugars, with foods that have the proper nutrients, our bodies will begin to heal themselves and our bodies will not crave like they did before. Remember, the body is an electrical fascinating machine, and it was created to flourish! Watch what it will do as we continue playing the game by our rules and with our strategy. I am the living proof of what I am telling you. I am back to my high school weight, feeling great and energetic. I did not focus on losing weight on my journey, but it was a delightful bonus. You can do this, and you will do this.

Lord, help us as we commit to living life Your way!

You don't need to take another pill or go on another diet of any kind if you don't want to. It's time to explore living life the way He predestined us to live. It promises greater results than we have ever experienced before through all the unhealthy and mostly unnatural things that profited you nothing but sickness and disease. You get to create your world through a game of whole ball or accept the world system game that we have been playing and losing.

Third rule: You will give your body some of the specific nutrients it's lacking. For example, I was diagnosed by the world with osteoporosis in my hips and spine. If you study this deficiency, it is caused by the density of bones and lack of calcium and the world says vitamin D. As I discovered the natural things my body would assimilate, I began to consume them as a part of my everyday food intake. Everything had to be plant based, with no starches, because I was reminded in Genesis that God gave me seed to plant and every tree with the leaves being for healing.

I introduced sea moss (a.k.a., Irish moss) into my daily routine. Look it up on Google and you can learn all about it. It carries 92 of the 102 nutrients and minerals that the body has, and the greatest is the one I need, calcium. It's virtually tasteless, so don't be afraid to try it. Another one is fresh dill, an herb that is high in calcium. I love the taste of dill, and it is helping this body come alive and vibrate at a higher frequency than ever before. Also, include fruit. For those the world has diagnosed with diabetes, for now you can only use certain fruits, but once your body is up and running at the capacity it was created to, you will be able to eat any of the fruits. *Please make sure if you are on prescribed medications that you seek the professional's opinion before going on this thirty-day journey.*

Most, if not all, the berries like blueberries, strawberries, raspberries, and elderberries, to name a few, are all high in nutrients and antioxidants. Try them one by one to see how your body responds. Our bodies will tell us what is good for it and what is not once it is awakened to its natural state. Fruits that have been tested and proven to be alkaline are small bananas or the burro/midsize banana, cantaloupe, cherries, currants, cherimoya (sugar apples), dates, and figs, to name a few to help you start your transition to a whole you.

If you're not sure about the pH of a certain food, you can buy a pH tester or you can always do a bit of research on the Internet. Always use two to three sources to confirm the pH. We want to get all fruits and veggies at or above pH 7. This means what? This means the fruit or vegetable is considered to be alkaline. Anything below pH 7 is acidic and can cause inflammation in the body, which can cause sickness and disease. Our cells have been compromised for a very long time but can recover given the right foods and help from the Creator and the entire heavenly host.

Calling all chefs! I am looking for some chefs who want to be food innovators by creating some tasty, healthy recipes to help others make an easier transition. Helping others will bring us so much pleasure. This was a great challenge when I started this journey because I could not find much information regarding plant-based food recipes. I became my greatest chef by putting these new foods together in creative ways. I know new healthy electrical plant-based restaurants are coming on the scene, which will help us and our children all to stay on this path forever. It's the God lifestyle that was given to us in the beginning. We are finding our way back. We will continue to grow in wisdom with an understanding of the alkaline world.

Most of us eat with our five senses fully active, so as you create your world or your game, be creative with high-energy foods and not just those that appeal to our senses. Remember, no starches for thirty days. I have found spelt, kamut, and teff flour, all of which are not starches. They are grains that are milled into flour but won't bind you or cause significant weight gain as enriched flour would. You can use them to make pancakes, waffles, fritters, etc. You will not miss the regular flours you grew up on, trust me.

God has created me to create, so I am creating new healthy recipes for foods that my body can assimilate. In the beginning, I didn't know what I was going to eat because everything was starch or sugar based. It was quite frustrating, but I could not turn back. I had the heavenly host cheering me on. I knew they were helping me to stay the course. One of the reasons for this book is because I wanted it to be the guide I didn't have. There were a few people I was told about who had vegan cookbooks, but only one resonated with me at the time because it was written by a vegan electrical chef. Find others who are following this path to help you get started or use the foods we've talked about and create your own recipes like I did. Don't say that you don't have time to cook healthy. I understand. I said the same thing initially. I don't know where the time came from, but it came. I know I had help from the unseen world. Preparation is an essential key. On your day off, prep your foods. Utilize YouTube videos that show you how to prepare smoothies. It makes it so easy to grab a baggie filled with our favorite fruits and green veggies and pop it in the blender, and we have a healthy breakfast filled with all the nutrients the cells need. We can do the same with salads, snacks, and desserts. I made it hard because I kept saying, "It's too hard." Who's up for a good challenge? The rewards make it worth the work.

Reflect

_____

_____

_____

_____

_____

_____

_____

_____

_____

_____

_____

_____

_____

_____

Electric U

CHAPTER 7

What's Your Motive?

What is your truth? What is the hidden agenda behind what you do? Do you skip meals to fit into that dress, those pants? Why do you do what you do?

Motive is a reason for doing something, especially one that is hidden or not obvious.

Let's examine what our motives are for wanting to lose weight. I had to ask myself this question. We must realize that many times, we do things for one reason that people can see but also an underlying reason usually no one can see. That is the driving force for why we do what we do, whether it is with good intentions or selfish intentions. We must ask ourselves this question and not be so hasty to answer it. Take some time and ponder this question, and write your answers down. Is it only selfish reasons? Perhaps you want to lose weight so you can look good and feel good about yourself. There is nothing wrong with those motives, right? Well, it depends. Does it stop there? Is it solely only about you? It is our human nature and how we have been conditioned that we only think about self. I was awakened to understand that my motives in the beginning for going on this journey were to help someone close to me only, and one day I heard, "Don't do it for someone else because when they don't accept it, you will be disappointed, discouraged, and all the other D places. You will most likely turn back to doing it the world's way. Do it because you need it just as much as anyone else may need it." I never thought long and hard about losing weight. It was never my motive or focus for any length of time, although I noticed the scale was on an upward trend. Weight loss, I understood, would be a single motive, but this was bigger than I ever imagined. I was given a driving force to break generational curses in my life that I learned were one of the culprits behind the way I was feeling in my body.

> The word *sin* means to miss. It doesn't
> mean to commit a wrong act; it
> simply means to miss, to be absent.

In sin did my mother conceive me. My journey is to discover what is missing, what is absent. We have to look at a bigger picture than just losing weight. Why are you unhappy with your weight? That will tell you there is something deeper than perhaps what you are looking at or what meets the eye. Weight is a symptom, not a root cause. When you find the root and uproot the hell of your past, the symptoms will disappear quicker than they appeared. Weight is not real. It is only a symptom of something bigger. The question is, do you want to uproot the hell of your past? That, my sisters and brothers, sons and daughters, is what should be our real motive or driving force. What I have found out is whatever the motive is that we may have for making the decision to start creating our game of whole ball. The Master Creator will change it if and when needed. I am being awakened daily to a hidden motive that He changes. There is no diet man can give you to uproot the hell of your past. Remember, cycles are real. Let's revisit these cycles that we talked about earlier.

Every facet of life has a cycle. We have the opportunity to break some of these cycles. First let's define the word cycle. Cycle is any complete round or series of occurrences that repeat or is repeated. Take health for example. "In sin did my mother conceive me." What does that mean? There are sin cycles of health conditions, education, finances, and even relationships that have been handed down from my mother to me, and the chain of life cycles continues. From as far back as we can go, we have missed something in our lives, something has been absent that has created these cycles in our lives. I believe the book of Genesis in the Bible shows us that His presence is what is missing from our lives. This has made it easy for us to live a life without Him, and it is what has set us up to live a life playing by the world's rules instead of our own.

Let's write our divorce papers to some life cycles and create our new vows.

We can start with saying, "Creator God, we surrender our will and our way and admit that we have lived unaware of the life You gave us. Lead us, and we will follow Your way. We want Your will for our lives. Thank You for all the good You have created for us. Thank You for opening our eyes to see Your way."

To get to place called "wholeness" requires our thinking to change. Most believe it's not possible or that we don't deserve it or the greatest one I hear all the time, "I *can't.*" You have what you say. If you are in any of those categories, then it's time for you to prophesy like *God* told Ezekiel. Speak to the dry bones, the dry places in your life and in your thinking until your thinking changes. You must be relentless! "As a man thinketh so is He" (Proverbs 23:7).

Let's pause for a moment and say, "God, give us a revelation of our thinking so we are provoked to change." The world calls this positive affirmation. God said, "Call those things that be not as though they were" (Romans 4:17). You have to be willing to write the vision and make it plain (Habakkuk 2:2). We know change is not easy, but I wonder why staying the same is. It's our choice— do we want easy, or do we want change? What do you think about yourself? Be as honest as you can. Take a few minutes and listen to the voice that is speaking right now. List all the "I can'ts" on a sheet of paper and then write all the "I cans" according to what God's word says. (Two blank pages have been provided.) Example: I can do all things through Christ who strengthens me. Now, let's make it practical. I can think like God thinks concerning my health, my weight, and what I eat daily. Today I make healthy eating choices. Today, I can park farther than ever before and walk to work, the grocery store, the mall, etc.

The key here is not to get upset with yourself if perhaps you miss your, "I *can*." Don't beat yourself up. The enemy would love to stop you before you even get started. Every day continue to speak it, and before you know it, you will have a change of mind and the manifestation will be in the here and now. Statistics say it takes twenty-one days to create a habit or change a bad habit. Go back and tear out the page that has all the "I cant's" and visualize the "I can." I believe and stand with you that you will do all things that pertain to the good of health for the body and soul.

Did you know speaking, sound, carries vibrations? As your vibration increases and gets higher, you will see more breakthrough, more victories in your life. In Joshua, they could not speak anything negative for seven days, and when they did speak, the sound in the words they spoke were powerful vibrations that were extremely high, causing the greatest mountain in their lives to crumble/collapse/come down. In order for that mind-set to collapse/crumble/come down, you are going to have silence the negative speaking to allow your words to carry higher vibrations, and then you will experience victory, enter your Promised Land, and have what you say! Lord Jehovah, let it *be*!

Reflect

Reflect

_____

_____

_____

_____

_____

_____

_____

_____

_____

_____

_____

_____

_____

_____

CHAPTER 8

Restoration of Wholeness

A time to restore us to wholeness does not mean it just happens overnight. I know we all wish it was that easy. In the book of Joshua, we see it was after the warrior the angel of the Lord went forth and eliminated the unseen foes that Joshua could go forth and victory was inevitable! When we read Joshua, we see he had to *go* and take the land from the enemies that were there. The land was their land, but it had been stolen from them and God had restored it to them. However, it required action on Joshua's and the Israelites' part. It was not just going to be brought to him and handed over on a silver platter. No, it required Joshua to *go* possess the land. *Go* means something was required of him. God said He has restored wholeness to us but we have to *go* get it. There is action required on our part. If you are sick in your body and it has caused you to be overweight, know that He has already provided your healing, but it requires you to *go* get it! How are you going to *go* get your healing? He will show you when you ask Him, "What do I need to do?"

Lord, we need to know how to *go* get our health that You gave back to us.

If you ask, He will show you. Just *go*! Go do the things He has told you to do. *Go.* Eat to live, and no more living to eat with your five senses. *Go* exercise. *Go* make right food choices. *Go* educate yourself on how and what to eat, how to exercise, etc.

I declare restoration in your life and that you will walk in wholeness in spirit, soul, and body, in Jesus's name! It was a journey of *go*ing for Joshua. When he got to the door of full restoration and manifestation, he had to circle that place for seven days. I believe it took time to get them to a place where they believed what God told them. We must also believe His promises for our lives. Everything has been given to us, health, wealth, and wholeness, and we can have it all. The one thing that the opposing forces use against us is fear. Fear had to be removed from the hearts of the people in the book of Joshua before they would *go* face the giants in that land. Giants represent those things that are big in our eyes that will hinder us from going forth in the way God tells us to *go*. It's a process, a journey to the place called wholeness, but we are assured He will get us there if we *go* (Joshua 5:13). We have the power and the authority to *go*.

We all understand keys unlock all kinds of doors. Well did you know keys can open kingdoms, which can represent resources for us? In Matthew 16:19, God said, "I have given you the keys to the kingdom of heaven." Keys represent our authority to open doors to kingdoms. What is a kingdom?

It is a political or territorial unit ruled by a sovereign, the eternal spiritual sovereignty of God or Christ. We have been given the key of authority over the kingdom, which represent us, our body, soul, and spirit. Have we given our keys to others, allowing them to rule over our bodies? Are we possibly allowing them to dictate what we should and should not eat and also, controlling other areas of our life like education, finances, even our children, just to name a few? Another area we will need to take authority over is our emotions. This area can be a huge hindrance to wholeness. Let's try to understand how emotions play a part in becoming whole.

On the path to wholeness, emotions will arise. Especially at certain times of the month for females, they rage a war in our members. Until the body has rid itself of the toxins, mainly starches and sugars, it will crave things that hurt the body and keep it a slave to what it wants, bondage. Remember, living to eat is not the way we want to live our lives. It takes time to change a pattern that has been in place for our entire life, so let's take one step at a time. Perhaps we can start by allowing ourselves to have the, "I just want it foods," once a day instead of whenever. The amazing thing I have realized on this journey is I am not alone, and I know it. There are spiritual forces with me, and they enable me to withstand the opposing forces of darkness. We can also refer to them as temptations. You will reach a point where the battle in your mind will be silenced, and when you are faced with that chocolate cake or candy, your mouth will no longer water. I know that's difficult to believe now, but I can assure you it will happen if you truly have set your face like flint toward wholeness. Isaiah 50:7 says, "LORD help me, I will not be disgraced. Therefore have I set my face like flint, and I know I will not be put to shame."

Pause, take a deep breath, and blow it out. Now let's say, "Lord, this is a mountain that I can't move, but I know You can cause it to crumble as I obey Your instructions, so let it be. I surrender." Let's begin to speak daily, "My emotions have no power against the spiritual forces that are with me!"

When wants rule our life, we become a slave to them. I am reminded of the story when Adam and Eve did not have to want for anything; however, they were introduced to wants that seemingly looked good to them. Adam and Eve chose what appealed to their senses, and it took them on a long journey to discover wants are not at all as good for you as they appear to be. Wants tend to have a beautiful array of color surrounding them. They can be bright and shiny to get our attention; however, they can put us into a place of bondage, which is what happened to Adam and Eve. It was too late when they realized want caused them to lose everything they had. The world of the wants and the want nots opened up and swallowed them. It took wholeness away and put them on an emotional rollercoaster of "I want that" and "I don't want that." I am convinced that is not the world I want any part of. I know it has been passed down to us; however, our eyes are being opened to what God gave us in the beginning, which is wholeness, oneness with *Him*. The world where He gives us the desires of our heart (Psalm 37:4), when He knows it's time, is where wholeness resides. He is the Captain of the ship of that world. My journey is dying to my "wants" and living the life of wholeness with Him. This is the place where all that is required of me is my obedience to His way and not my way.

Let go and trust Him to be the King of your kingdom, body, and soul (mind, will, emotions). It's a new path given to us. The choice is mine and yours. "Choose you this day whom you will serve" (Joshua 24:15).

Nuggets of Truth/Food for Thought

Did you know? Our bodies have millions of living cells. Living cells are a small form of life, but they perform all the biological functions in the body. They absorb our nourishment, and they breathe and release toxins. When cells cannot function in this way, they can become ill and only reproduce unhealthy cells, causing sickness and disease.

Hybrids are plants, foods, or animals that are created when you mix two different species. This comes from the hands of man. They change the genetic integrity. It becomes a starch, acid-based plant.

Nonhybrid food means it have its full genetic integrity intact. For example, organic grapes are not seedless. If the grapes do not have seeds, they are a process of sterilization. Stay away from them. Seedless watermelons are also hybrids. They are combining new species that have been genetically changed. They tell us they want to make it convenient for us, but the real intent is greed. When have you known this world system not to have a hidden agenda?

Why are they changing our foods? The answer is simple: for financial gain. To create something new is very empowering. However, we have to understand that the cross-breeding culture of plants can be detrimental to our body.

Reflect

_____

_____

_____

_____

_____

_____

_____

_____

_____

_____

_____

_____

_____

_____

CHAPTER 9

Are Old Habits Hard to Break?

There is a saying we often tell ourselves: "Old habits are hard to break." Well, that has been true in the past, but my saying now is, "Habits are being broken every day in me." Every habit that has not brought me to a wealthy place, spirit, soul, and body is being annihilated! There is no place for poverty, lack, or bankruptcy in my spirit, soul, or body. My focus is to be a sharp shooter. I will spot those habits that have been in my life for a long time and have gone unnoticed and demolish them.

Somewhere in our minds, we have been conditioned to think it's okay to let old habits rob us. Perhaps we are oblivious of them stealing, killing, and destroying our lives. They are our target now, and we aim to kill on the spot! Let's create a natural target on a sheet of paper, and every day we aim and shoot at it. Make labels of all the old habits you have not been able to break in your life. Take the paper with all of those old habits, and tape or roll it onto a small piece of aluminum foil and say, "Thank You, Lord, this old habit is broken." Daily throw it at the bull's-eye. Let's practice daily, because we know it's not so easy to hit the bull's-eye on a target in reality, but with practice, we will do it! Let's have some fun on this journey to wholeness. Place a target in your bathroom on a mirror or a place you frequently go every day multiple times. As a man thinketh, so is he. We are visual people, so it is important that we get a visual of overcoming obstacles in our life. It's a simple but powerful challenge. Perhaps it sounds silly to you, but if it works, it won't be silly to you. Get creative, and make up your game that will create a visual for you. Every day we see it and say it, our mindsets are shifting. Yes, it may take some time, but it's okay. We have been sick for a very long time. To come out of this place will take time. We have to develop patience, love, compassion, and forgiveness along the way. I believe God has brought us to this place and He will get us to our destination, which is wholeness. Let's enjoy the journey. Make sure you journal your path daily. Trust me, you won't recall all the details when you get to the finish line and look back. How often do we try to look back to recall how we got to a certain destination, and it seems the details fade away? If you write them, you will be able to share with others. It's important as we learn what works for our bodies to share with others our successes. Continuing on our journey to wholeness, let's look at more truths.

Let's open our hearts to receive truth even if it challenges us in ways that make us uncomfortable. Ponder these questions for a while before you give an answer.

1. Are you willing to risk it all and leave everything behind to get to wholeness?
2. If you knew better, would you do better?
3. The truth will set you free. But suppose the truth did not look so good?
4. What will you do if you know the truth is not pretty?

The ugly truth we are facing concerning many if not all facets of our life is that greed is leading the motives of most, if not all of what is being done in the area of food, the health industry, etc. Suppose your weight gain is directly related to greed, and I don't mean your greed. Suppose what you eat has been altered to cause you to eat and eat and eat, which creates not only obesity but sickness and disease. The goal that is being achieved at our expense is not pretty. Your cravings have been created by greed. It is not your fault. We have been tricked or conditioned to believe the lie that we should live to eat. If you knew better, would you do better? The answer may be, "Maybe or maybe not." Our cravings that have been created are not easy to break. It's like an addiction, which we all have experienced in some way. Maybe we have been affected perhaps by a friend or family member who has suffered from an alcohol or drug addiction. We know it is extremely difficult to break because those who created it, their motivation is and was greed. They have assured the ingredients were strong enough to keep the addict coming back for more. Well, they have done the same thing with food, only it's legal. The vast majority who are benefiting from our addictions is earth shattering. If only we could see behind the scenes what is really going on, we would be astounded. Lord Jesus, we need the greater forces to be with us for sure if we are going to be able to escape the claws of the enemy! The scripture says, "The thief cometh but to steal, kill and destroy." This thief is the food they are giving us to consume that appeals to our five senses. Some of these foods are literally stealing, killing, and destroying us daily. God said He came that we may have life and have it more abundantly. Did you know that life comes by way of death? Isn't that a strange truth? To have the life He promised, we will have to walk a death walk. Interesting, wouldn't you say? Well most of us would say well Jesus died, and He did it for us. Yes, that's true; He did it to give us power to do it. We are required to die daily to the things of this world. Remember I asked if you would do better if you knew better? I said maybe or maybe not. This is why. You may want to do better, but there are great things put in place to assure even if you know better you will not do better. Why? Because no one wants to die. The will of man to live is ancient, meaning very old and strong. It takes dying to your will to eat to live. Everywhere you turn, the focus is on what you eat because they know everyone eats with their eyes and then with their mouth. The appeal is to your emotions, which is a biggie that we talked about earlier. It is definitely a sacred cow! Everyone wants to feel good and full and satisfied, and those who benefit from this truth know it and are capitalizing off of that truth every day! Now ask yourself, if you knew better, would you do better?

When I started this journey, I knew there were things I did not think I could live without, but I can honestly say I was very surprised how easy it was. I knew I was going to need greater forces than myself for this journey. Little did I know midway in He would show me this journey started long before I agreed to it. Years earlier I noticed I was losing the taste for certain things I had eaten all my life, and I could not explain why. All I knew was I did not have a taste for them anymore. Now I realize He chose the journey for me and not I for it, and therefore, all I needed to do was consent, choose it mentally and surrender to it when it knocked at my door to come in and live with me. When I surrendered to it, I did not tell anyone, just in case I could not stay the course. Months into the journey, as I changed what I ate, when I ate, and how I ate, I found, to my surprise, that I no longer had the feeling of being hungry. I thought to myself, *This is strange. Why am I not hungry? I have to eat.* As I stayed on the path, I began to receive understanding. What I now understand is that starchy foods cause you to crave more starchy food, just like sugar addicts crave more sugar. The artificial starchy foods and sugars are out of my diet, and now, I no longer crave those foods. Now I understand why the majority of the foods we eat and love are starch based. That one element alone will keep you hungry! Wow, unbelievable! I asked, "Why, Lord?"

Nothing happens without His consent, as difficult as that is to believe. He said, "All things will work together for our good." All of our experiences, good or seemingly bad, will bring us back to understand that without God, we can't do anything. We are nothing without the Creator. At some point on the path, we will come to trust Him in all things pertaining to our lives. We began with the Creator, and we will ultimately end with the Creator. The ugly truth that I had to come to grips with is the spirit of greed is ferocious. We can't blame those who are benefiting; it's not their fault either. We have been victims of a broken system. The more you get, the more you want and are allowed to have, with strings, debt, obesity, low self-esteem, and so many others. We need to understand this perpetrator we named greed. Whether it is money, food, or other things, you will always want more. You will never be able to say, "I am complete. I don't want for anything." Greed will not allow anyone to be satisfied or content. Oh sure, we all experience a few moments of pleasure where we may have said that, but the moment fled quickly. We all are exposed and vulnerable to greed, so we can't be judgmental. Our goal is to understand how the spirit operates so we can escape the claws of this enemy. It won't be easy, but it is possible.

Food for Thought
Did You Know?

The native plant structure that came with the planet has 102 minerals, and they are easy for your body to assimilate. They become one with your body. Could this be why God said in Genesis, Ezekiel, and Revelation, "The trees/leaves are for the healing of the nations"? He made them electrical, and we are electrical also. In the beginning He gave spirit man seed and put seed on the earth to reproduce after its kind.

Acid interrupts our harmonious flow; it robs us of our energy. Starch converts into carbonic acid. Get ready to use the keys He gave you.

Greed is the same as gluttony, self-indulgence, craving, longing, wish, passion. The definition of greed is intense and selfish desire for something, especially wealth, power, or food.

He without sin can cast the first stone. We all are targets/prey of this enemy called greed. We may not have benefited as much as those responsible for the food industry giving us hybrids for their gain, but we are culprits as well. I don't know about you, but I no longer wish to play their game or contribute to their pockets continuing to get fat. I have taken a huge step out of the game, and I tell you, it is so rewarding. Are you ready to give up adding to their increase?

Reflect

_____

_____

_____

_____

_____

_____

_____

_____

_____

_____

_____

_____

_____

Electric U

CHAPTER 10

Building Time—a Reconstruction of Our Body/Our Health

It is a time to build a fortified kingdom/body. How do I accomplish such a task, one may ask? Well first it is necessary to ignite some things in us. Maybe a good place to start is to look at where the heat is coming from. Is it the roof, what is at the top? What is the number one thing that is wreaking havoc in your life, the one thing you don't feel you can live without? That is where the roof is on fire. That is where the heat is coming from. We must target that first. Will it be easy? Of course not. Life is never easy and He did not promise it would be, but He promised to be with us always even until the end (Deuteronomy 31:6). Our assurance is we can do all things through Him that strengthens us (Philippians 4:13). It's important to take out the top, the chief culprit, first, and then rebuild. Is it sugar or starch? Put them in order, the greatest to the least. Mine was bread; I had to eat it every day or I would have some kind of reaction. I could never get enough. My addictive

68

behavior inherited from generations causes me to not be able to control things I really like. What's yours? Just the thought of it sets you on fire, right? I really do understand, and I have empathy for addicts. Whatever sets you on fire must be your target. I said, "God, I can't do this and I know I can't, but You have my permission to do it through me. I am willing to let it go." Then I paused and said, "I think I am ready, but everything in me is screaming, I can't let go.'" I knew I had to, but nothing in me wanted to. Well, after the pity party, I geared up for the battle. I was ready to go through withdrawals or whatever it took to free me from the clutches of this food opponent. Once I set my spirit, soul (mind, will, and emotions), and body like flint, I dove into it. One week went by, and I said, "Oh, wow, I made it!" No oatmeal, no cinnamon toast, no sweet potato, no eggs, no *bacon*, no sausage, none of my favorite things that I consumed daily. Wow, I could not believe I'd gone a week without any of them. The next week, I didn't waver and on and on, week after week, month after month. I was amazed. I know it was done not by might nor by power, but by *His* Spirit. What I had devoured for *years*, now gone! That was definitely unbelievable to me. Around the second month, I reached the plateau. I realized I was no longer experiencing hunger for any of the things I longed for the majority of my life. Over fifty years I'd eaten this way, and in two months, it was gone! I did not understand how this happened. He showed me that starchy and sugary foods cause cravings. They will never be satisfied, just like greed. If you remove them for a certain length of time until you reach the plateau, you will be free from their claws. Now the body can do what it was created to do—begin the healing process. The body was so violated by those things that I gave it that it could not do what it was created to do. I started noticing things, my sight was clearing up (not my physical eyesight, but my spiritual eyesight was giving me the ability to see truth in a way I never saw before), and my hips and joints and back and shoulders were not hurting. The bottom of my feet were not paining me, and I was not getting the sharp pains in my toes. I was astounded to say the least. Could this be true? Was what I was eating preventing me from being whole the way God created me? Yes, I can emphatically say yes! I am living proof. Everything we put in our mouths has a negative or positive reaction on the body, whether we notice (can see) it or not. It is wreaking havoc in some way on the body.

Chaos comes in our lives when an acidic substance enters the body. When it is removed, love peace will enter in the body, and we will see clearly. I could not see what I was eating was offending my body. I thought sweet potatoes were good for me, but not understanding it is a hybrid starchy base, therefore the body will not assimilate it. We have been conditioned to believe things that are not true for us according to our DNA, our cellular disposition. Starch, I now understand, converts into carbonic acid. If nature does not produce the substance, it will cause inflammation in the body. What God gave us to consume is starchless foods. The difficulty is finding the things that are true to nature. We understand that nowadays everything has been altered in some way. However, God is leading us to what to eat and what not to eat. Studying and asking lots of questions is a must on this journey.

We are going to have to utilize Google like never before. We can't be lazy and spend hours in front of a television. That is filling us for the most part with false hope and feeding our emotions. I began to get up early and spend what I call time in the "stillness space" or quiet time with my Creator, to fill me with what I needed for that day. I gave up television for a while and used that time to learn as much as I can about this journey He has chosen for me. I also find time at the end of the day when the house is quiet, which allowed me to study, listen to videos, and research on Google and the Hebrew Bible, in an effort to discover truth. If my body feels this way by just eliminating starches and sugars and certain meats, like pork and beef, out of my diet, there has to be truth in what we are putting in our bodies that is reaping havoc in our bodies. I am sharing because I found this truth, and I believe this vital key was not just given to me for me, but for others, like my grands and generations to come, to know the truth and have the opportunity to choose truth over what has been given to us. I don't believe I chose to go on this journey. I believe it was chosen for me, and I said yes. Now I am the recipient of all the benefits I am sharing with others.

A twelve-year-old girl, whose name is unknown, wrote this poem after seeing and hearing her mother be treated naturally of a disease in her body, and she was taught what caused her mother disease.

Starch and blood will cause a
flood that floods the brain

That brings the pain that
makes her blame.
—Arthur Unknown

I thought it so powerfully captures the truth of what happens to us when we consume these things that are not natural and the body can't assimilate, causing excessive weight gain, sickness, and diseases in our temple, our kingdom, which is our body that we have been given the keys to rule over.

Food for thought: an eagle knows how to make a nest, and it was never taught. It's coded in the DNA. What's coded in your DNA related to what should and should not be eaten?

Theory

The composition of life has a base of carbon, hydrogen, and oxygen. The things that are made by nature contain these three things and will assimilate in the body. If they don't have the three things, they are acid substance and should not be consumed. The body will not assimilate it, and therefore it will cause sickness and disease in the body.

Reflect

_____

_____

_____

_____

_____

_____

_____

_____

_____

_____

_____

_____

_____

_____

_____

_____

Electric U

CHAPTER 11

We Are the Apple of His Eye!

Do you truly understand you are uniquely and wonderfully made and there is no one else with your fingerprint, which makes you incredibly special? Take a deep breath slowly, release it, slowly exhaling, and ponder how God took the time to create you. Do you realize how special you are that the Creator would make you in His image and likeness? This is a powerful truth that we read but don't take the time to become *one* with this truth. We have been beaten down so much by life experiences until we never were able to really breathe this truth in our very fiber of our being. We often look at ourselves in the mirror and see all the negative things that we don't like about ourselves, like nose too big, lips too big, hair too short, too tall, too fat, etc., and some even spending lots of money to make the exterior look perfect by the world's standards. We can all write a book of the negative things about our self, but the positive things would not reach a page. But think for a few minutes about how God views His creation. He wants to be *one* with you.

He says you are fearfully and wonderfully made in His image and His likeness. We are oneness/wholeness with our Creator, living and breathing in us the very core and fiber of who we are in *Him*. We have been so disconnected from that truth, so now it seems like that is the lie, and the truth is, we are these broken, sinful people that God has left to fend for ourselves. Have you ever looked at a flower, like an orchid, and how beautiful it is in all of its many beautiful, vibrant colors? Well, we can see the beauty in it. Why can't we see the beauty in ourselves? You are that orchid, that beautiful, full of radiant color butterfly that we all admire, which I have heard someone say they are "flowers with wings." The same God who took His time and created the flowers is the same God who created you and me. Our perspective of ourselves has to change. You have to see yourself the way God sees you with all your so-called imperfections that we have been told day in and day out we have. Stand in the mirror and say, "I am beautiful! I am incredibly special; there is no one else in the whole world like me!" Our self-esteem plays a direct role on our bodies and souls (mind, will, emotion). If you don't think highly of yourself, then you will not treat your body like the kingdom temple He created it to be. You will abuse it and neglect it and treat it the way you think of it. Our image of ourselves is directly related to whether we walk in the wholeness He destined us for. It is time to turn our thoughts of our self into positive thoughts. It is time you see yourself the way God sees you. He provided everything you need to stay healthy and beautiful, strong and vibrant. We have to take back what was stolen from us—yes, our self-worth, self-esteem, respect, appreciation, value, and honor. We must know we are whole, spirit, soul, and body! He created us whole, so it is achievable to live and breathe in this truth. No longer complain about the body He gave you. Let's do something about what we don't like instead of complaining about it. I don't mean to pay someone to change it. If you love yourself, treat yourself with the respect you so deserve. Learn about this fascinating machine, and love it enough to give it what it needs, not what it wants.

For as he thinks in his heart,
so is he (in behavior).
—Proverbs 23:7

Going to a place you have never been before can be scary to us sometimes, but if we want to go to new places and experience new things, we must be willing to *go*! Evict *fear,* and *go* to the unknown places. You have to understand you are not the driver; He is, so we are assured to be in good hands and will get there safely. He is with us as we embark upon new territory. He is always there to help when it gets too challenging. As we get a true picture of the wealth that has been entrusted to us, let's learn as much as possible about this wealthy person He created us to be. We are powerful, and He has crowned us with His glory. There is nothing too difficult for us, because the Greater One lives in us.

As we take a look at what this incredible machine called our body is made of, we are told by science, who has studied this fascinating machine we call the body, that it is 70 percent water. Another allegory is hidden here, which is, water representing the Spirit, so for me that means a lot. It means you are more spirit than you are a natural human being. I learned I was not drinking enough water, so I decided to increase my intake, and to my amazement, on my first day, I was taken on a spiritual journey. Yes, I went to the bathroom a lot, but more importantly, I had so many dreams, and the important part was I was able to recall them in detail, which I had not been able to do most of the time. This means that water also increases our vibrations. It is electric. Try it; don't take my word for it. Drink as close to a gallon as you can, and record the results. It not only cleanses our cells, but it awakens and strengthens our spirit man, which causes the spirit man to take flight, ascending to higher heights. It increases your frequency to vibrate on another level.

Natural foods that God made and good water are essential to this journey to wholeness. If you are fighting an infirmity in your body, double or triple your water intake. Try to use PH water, preferably 8 or higher, until you rid the body of toxins that have invaded your cells, causing them to be compromised. I promise you will see an immediate difference in day two. I have not only found this to be true for me but for others as well. You will feel better quicker, which means your recovery is well on its way. It may take weeks before you fully recover, depending on how much the cells have been compromised and the level of mucus that has accumulated in the body. Don't give up. Be consistent. I believe God created this body to heal itself, and it will when we give it what the Creator created for it. God saw the end from the beginning, so He knew "flesh man" would leave His presence and be faced with sickness and disease. Wholeness is a place where no sickness or disease can enter the body or soul (mind, will, emotion). If you look around at all the sickness and disease, you may feel this is not possible. We all feel at times this is so far from our reach. I believe today more than ever before we are being awakened to the truth of who we are, and that, my friend, is the beginning of the journey to wholeness. Yes, it's a place most of us can only dream about but have not ever been, but I want to go, so I say daily, "Take me there, Lord." I believe I am well on my way. Yes, it has taken me years. It feels like a century, but I am now well on my way. All my life I have felt like I have been fighting sickness of some kind, and now to begin to rid my body of it feels oh so good. We are well on our way by taking even one step in this direction. Sounds too easy to be true. Well, it's true and it is easy, because we are not alone. He is driving, so we are sure to get there safely. Easy does not mean easy in the way we are accustomed to it. Easy now means God is showing us the way and causing us to see that help is with us now. Becoming awakened to these truths is a huge step that makes the journey easy. Our struggle has been because we were working in our strength and felt alone.

Nugget of Truth

Every cell is made up of a different structure a different mineral. The brain is made up of copper and carbon, the bone calcium, and the blood iron. Let's find the foods that contain these minerals and eat them daily, comprehending you are eating to live!

Food for Thought

We have been divorced from that which is natural and married to that which is unnatural. Using this allegory, let's plan some beautiful weddings. We are the beautiful brides marrying (becoming one) with our Creator that created us.

Nugget of Truth

Iron is by far the most important mineral, because it is electric and magnetic. Iron is important because it draws all of the minerals needed for the body to thrive. The iron the body will assimilate is plant based. Artificial iron will bind us; however, plant irons will not. This is how you know it's one with your body arrangement.

When acid enters the human body, it disrupts all systems. It interrupts our harmonious flow, robbing us of our energy. Iron that is consistent with the body has carbon, hydrogen, and oxygen. If we look for a plant that has dominant iron, carbon, there is infinity—chemical infinity. When there is infinity, there is assimilation.

Reflect

_____

_____

_____

_____

_____

_____

_____

_____

_____

_____

_____

_____

_____

_____

CHAPTER 12

New Life New Day

Have you taken a step? Are you embracing new life? It's a new day for us—an awakening to embracing our new body as it is being transformed. I am loving this new life as I get closer to wholeness. My thoughts are getting clearer. I am feeling so much better, but I realize I have just begun. I am taking it very slow on this journey—one step at a time. I have come to understand that I was born sick. All of us were born sick, so it is not something that will change overnight. I also know that most of what we are eating that we know as food have been tampered with in some way by man, which is contributing to our bodies being in the condition they are in. Hybrids and GMOs are everywhere. Do we know what the original versions of the foods we are eating now were? It's pretty complex for sure, so we need all the help we can get from heaven to guide us to what is best for the fascinating machine God made that we call our bodies. Well, the good thing is I am not where I was, and I am not where I ultimately want to be. However, I am well on my way. I have made some drastic leaps toward my goal. I can feel the changes in my body, and that assures me I am on the right track. I am playing the new game, and I am winning every day. I don't look at the days I miss the mark. I just keep my eyes on the prize, which is wholeness. Each day I set goals, but not without the understanding that if I don't meet or supersede the goal for the day, it's okay. There is always tomorrow. I have taken the pressure off myself to achieve everything put in front of me. I will take some steps toward my goal, but if I don't make it, there will be no backlash from me or anyone else. Thank You, Lord. This journey is a personal journey that involves the Creator, me, myself, and I. It's important to take everyone else out of the equation. I heard it said before, "Difficulties are opportunities to show our greatness." As we draw closer to the place called wholeness, greatness peeks out and gets brighter and clearer to obtain. I took another leap that I thought was impossible, and that was to go a day without meat. Yes, a day. It's a step toward the goal. I have eaten meat two to three or more times every day of my life unless I was fasting, which is another subject we will discuss later. I discovered the food industry is not considering what is good for me and how meats are hybrid, meaning they are altered by man. I know that is shocking to most—at least it was for me. Did you know a horse is complete? It was made by God. A jackass is complete, made by God. Well, where did a mule come from? It's a hybrid. They made a horse mate with a jackass, and what we got was a mule. Do your research. You may be surprised about what you learn. Man is interfering with God's creation. A mule is half of each of the original animals created by God.

God is awakening us to the truth for a greater purpose than we may understand at this point. What is coming to our tables is sickness and disease. If we don't understand that greed is embedded in everything man is creating, by the time the next generation's babies grow up, they won't have a clue what they are eating. Sickness and disease are inevitable for them in some way, shape, or form. Their only hope is to go back to the beginning of the foods God created for us to consume. The herbs are for the healing of the body (Genesis 1:29). And the leaves of the trees are for the healing of the nation (Revelation 22:2). This is where the key to living life to the fullest is hidden. My quest is to teach my grands how to make wise choices for their health so when they are old, they will know how to keep their temples healthy and whole, and hopefully it will be easier for them to stay the path than it is for my generation and my children's generation.

Proverbs 15:17 says, "Better is a dinner of herbs where love is, than a stalled ox and hatred therewith."

Did You Know?

Hybrid is the crossing of two products/animals with another that would not normally come together.

GMO or genetically modified organism can be defined as organisms (i.e., plants, animals, or microorganisms) in which the genetic material (DNA) has been altered in a way that does not occur naturally by mating and/or natural recombination.

Eat to live or eat to die is my choice, and it was looking in the face of my forefathers cheering me on. With their help, I chose to step on a new path different from any I had known. Was it difficult? Yes, but the alternative was to continue to eat to die like everyone in my family was doing. How would I expect anything different if I did what they did? I would most likely die like they died, with diabetes, arthritis, cancer, etc. I looked in their faces and knew I was given an opportunity to escape the way they died, which was with sickness and diseases. We all need to look in the faces of our ancestors and choose a new path different from any of our ancestors were able to do. The information and the help did not come for them but it has come to our generation, and so it is our responsibility to heed the opportunity afforded us. They perhaps were seeds sown so we could have the opportunity to receive the harvest. The question is what we do with the information afforded to us now. Do we want to continue our lives saying, "I can't," or do we look to the hills from whence our help cometh and tell "self" we can do it and we will do it? I have come to understand since I have begun this journey that there is a threshold, and once we cross it, we will sail, with wind beneath our sail thrusting us forward. The challenge is getting to and crossing that threshold. The war is real, and it is the war between the old you and the new you. The new you wants to make changes, but the old you is fighting to prevent the new one from going on this new path. The voices speaking in your ears are so loud, telling you what you can't do and what you should do. Many give up on the journey before getting to the threshold because of the war that is going on inside them. More and more people, more now than ever before, are winning the war, so it is achievable! I crossed that threshold, and I am sailing now. Nothing is difficult. The voices have been silenced in me. You can do it. Just choose to walk through the door and let the battle begin. If we look at the journey as too great of a challenge, then it will be just that, but if we look at the journey as achievable, no sweat we will obtain it. It's all about our perspective. It's time to look at life, food, and health differently. Don't be afraid to enter into the battle with the intent to win. The next time you put anything in your mouth, think about what it will do for you. Will it bring you to the place called wholeness, or will it bring you to a place called sickness and disease? We know the flesh is weak but the spirit man is willing, and that is why we have to build the spirit man up strong to help us not give in to the flesh man's (human part of us) desires. I recommend introducing alkaline foods into your diet as much as possible because it will give the new you strength and change your taste buds. Remember, our taste buds have been robbed, but we can and will get them back.

I know it feels like eating like this will rob us of the pleasures of life, but no, not at all. You might say what I said—what will I eat at a restaurant, or when invited to someone's house? Don't worry, in the beginning you will be tempted and you will give into the temptations, and that's okay. You will come to a place where your taste buds will change and you will not be tempted. The "new you" will not want any of the old foods. I know it seems impossible, but it happens over time. Now, if I am invited out to someone's home and I don't know if they will have food that I like, I eat before I leave home. This way I am not pressured to eat what I know will not benefit my body. We have been given an opportunity to create new pleasures of life. We are creators, so we get to create new recipes using healthier ingredients that we can enjoy, that are alkaline, and that our bodies can assimilate. This is a new perspective.

Creator Lord God, help us get to and cross the threshold. We need Your power to not give in and give up to the cravings that have had their claws in us for too long. Break the chains so we can go free to be all You have destined for us to be in the earth. Our health is our wealth.

Reflect

_____

_____

_____

_____

_____

_____

_____

_____

_____

_____

_____

_____

_____

_____

Electric U

CHAPTER 13

A Better You

You no longer have to choose to eat the things that are robbing us of our God given health. We can choose the wealthy place and not look back. I am truly grateful for this new life I have been afforded to live. Feeling Great! Make the choice today to eat to live! Don't die to eat any longer. It's time to be a better *you*.

What I want everyone to know is what I was awakened to know. It's not your fault. We are being awakened to realize we are all born addicts. It's not our parents' fault, as I have said many times; it's a system that we all were born into. My parents were both addicts, and their parents were also. It was not their fault or ours. We were made addicts by the society in which we live. At some point, it seems society stopped loving people and started loving money. Money is ruling. Everything is based on how much money we can make. Is it surprising? No, because the Bible says the love of money is the root of all evil (1 Timothy 6:10). We are all products of this evil and not by choice. We were removed from the pure and clean life our ancestors once enjoyed, where everything in that environment was good and everything we needed was provided. But we were at some point put in another environment that was a toxic environment. We are being brought back to the original life God intended for us to live. It's a choice we will have to choose. I believe as we continue to live healthier lifestyles, we will see everything through a new lens. Everything will get clearer when we let go of our acidic diets and turn to an alkaline lifestyle. This is the pure and clean, and they enjoyed it in the garden in the beginning of time that we read about in the Bible. We have to return to this lifestyle if we want to enjoy the healthier life that has been afforded to us. I believe man will continue to bring foods to us that we have not seen or heard of, and it will taste very good to our palates but will bring sickness and disease to our bodies. What God created is alkaline, which is electrical for the electrical bodies that He gave us. Man can never duplicate what God created. He gave man herb/seed, which will reproduce after its own kind. Man is altering God-created foods, and they are causing sickness and diseases in our bodies. The challenge becomes how to know the difference between acidic and alkaline. There are studies that have been performed on the different fruits and veggies we are consuming, and they have found that anything with a pH of 7 or below is acidic and anything above 7 is alkaline. Foods high on the pH scale promote the transmission and integrity of the human body (electrical system). Acidic foods low on the pH scale are detrimental to the body. They cause dysfunction and weaken our bodies. We have computers that are able to give us information at a stroke of a key. Do your research. Your body deserves it! God gave you rule over it. You are the beautiful garden

He planted in this earth, and He wants you to flourish. Tools that may help you when you choose to eat to live are on the next pages. Study to show yourself approved unto God (2 Tim 2:15). Your body will thank you. The more you learn, the more empowered you are to do what is right for the electrical machines we call the body. The answers are available, but we have to search for them. They will not be handed to us. Ask lots of questions, and read as much as possible. I will show some of the things I have learned during my countless hours of studying what are electrical and what are the best foods to consume. It's not always easy to do what is right, and we often don't choose what is right. However, we must not ever give up. If you were diagnosed with a life-threatening disease, would it make it easier to choose what is right, if it would give you more time in this earth? Well think of it that we are all one step away from that diagnosis if we don't make some changes concerning our health. Most of what is in grocery stores and the restaurants is not there for our benefit. They are there to make money. Their efforts are put into how they can get us to buy as much sugary and processed foods as possible. Think about this for a moment. Everything is geared toward triggering your taste buds that drives you to crave more of what will not benefit your body.

Cravings are not easily broken because what we are eating is the reason we have the cravings in the first place. It's like a person on drugs who can't stop doing the drugs. What has to happen is to remove the person from the drugs, normally for a certain length of time to get him or her strong enough to break the craving. Fasting works similarly. It is one of the most effective ways to break the cravings because, you take away the foods that are causing the cravings for a period of time, and your body will begin healing itself. There are many types of fasting that we can choose, but always consult a physician if you are on medications.

I am a living testimony this works because, years ago I was addicted to bread. I ate it every day and multiple times a day for years. Every year my church would go on a forty-day fast. One year, the pastor's instructions were to give up something you really love for forty days. Immediately, bread flashed before me. I quickly dismissed it and said, "I will give up television." Then I think the pastor heard my thoughts, because he said, "Make sure it's something you really love." I gave in and said, "Okay, I will give it up for forty days, and perhaps I will be able to control it after the forty days." The battle began, and it was literally a war in my members physically. I went through withdrawals for weeks. I had headaches and sweats, and my mouth watered every time I saw bread. I could not go down that aisle in the grocery store because I would literally get the shakes. I now have empathy for drug addicts because of what I walked through during those forty days. Many times I said, "I can't do it." The mental war was bad, but the physical war was greater. Only with God's help did I make it through the forty days. To my utter surprise, on day forty-one, I could not wait to get the bread. I ate it and realized it did not taste the same, and I was so disappointed. I did not want to give it up. I only wanted to control it. God knew that was not possible, so the taste was totally taken away. My body no longer craved it because it was healed. My taste buds completely changed. I learned a lot from that experience. They put certain ingredients in breads that make you addicted. Our bodies will heal if given the chance. Fasting has been proven to work for me and countless others. If you are wondering if I eat bread now, the answer is occasionally, but it still does not taste like it did when I was addicted. Fasting is not just good to break any addictions, but it is just as good or better spiritually. Your spirit will be stronger. You will not be the same you after fasting. I won't say it will take forty days to break an addiction, but fasting any time will give your body the opportunity to heal itself and change your taste buds and become strong spiritually. Your light will definitely be brighter. As I always like to say, don't take my word for it. Try it for yourself. Start with three days and then go to seven days and then twenty-one days. One important factor in fasting is to drink plenty of good water. Remember, your body is made up of 70 percent water. Do research to see the benefits of fasting, and you may be convinced to try it. When you try taking something away, add something healthy that will aid your body in becoming whole faster—for example, removing cookies and adding fruit of choice. Taking away artificial sugar and replacing it with natural sugar the body can process easier is how we change to a healthier lifestyle. Change your diet and you change your life. Life changers, let's change our diets.

Reflect

_____

_____

_____

_____

_____

_____

_____

_____

_____

_____

_____

_____

_____

Electric U

CHAPTER 14

Busy Minded vs. Stillness

Have you ever tried to be in the moment without your mind wandering? Have you ever walked into a room and realized you did not know how you got there or forgot what you went into the room for? Well, I am guilty of both. I realize that my mind was not in the moment even though my body was moving. Many of us don't even realize our minds are always busy. Try being in the moment in everything you do, and you will probably realize how challenging this is. Our lives are steady on go, seemingly 24-7. The only time we stop is when we go to sleep, and even that seems to be robbing us of dreams. The moment we are conscious of being awoken, our minds are on the go. I meet people all the time who tell me they don't dream, and I tell them, "Yes you do, but you don't recall them." We are spirit beings, and God communicates through dreams now, as we see throughout the Bible. Our busy lives are robbing us of our spiritual inheritances. This is the wealthy place where all our treasures are. Remember, we are made in God's image and likeness. We have a spirit that is alive. It may be sleeping, but it can be awakened. Knowing the truth is one way we awake our spirit man. Food is the one I concentrate on for becoming whole.

As we are on the journey to wholeness, it will help us if we spend time being still. I replace the word *meditation* with the word *stillness*. Meditation for many is too difficult to achieve. I find the stillness place seems more achievable, because I created it. I have found this place is packed with power, and it is available. However, we will have to fight the opposing forces that await us when we attempt to get in this space. The mind will oppose us by going on its on journey the moment we set our minds to be still. Thoughts will come faster than you can imagine, taking you on a journey. The key again is persistence. The benefits far outweigh the challenges. We have been busy minded for so long we don't realize it is a problem and that it is robbing us of our inheritance. Let's be mindful of what we are doing every moment. We have to learn to fully embrace each moment with our full awareness being drawn to that moment. For example, if you are talking to a friend, fully engage in what is being said at that moment. I am guilty of being not fully engaged when in a conversation. The mind is always busy, but it's time to slow it down because it is robbing us of treasures that are priceless.

Visions await us in the stillness space—wisdom and understanding, counsel and might, knowledge and the reverential fear of God. Wealth and riches abide in this space, and they all await us to receive their power-packed benefits in our life.

Scientific studies have been documented of the benefits of what they call meditation. You can do the research for yourself. How it affects the brain's frontal coherence is interesting. The unity and cohesiveness that occurs is beyond our complete understanding. I recommend you spend some time reading about the benefits documented by research. Perhaps it will assist you to pursue this space for yourself.

Be still and know that I am God (Psalm 46:10). It is in the place of stillness that we have the opportunity to know our Creator. It's in our stillness that our Creator is exalted. It behooves us to pursue this place with all that is in us because greatness awaits us there.

Prayer is an excellent tool many have been taught, but it is different from stillness. I believe it is on a different vibration or level than we have understood. In prayer we have been taught to talk to God, but in stillness we don't talk. We are still and wait for God to talk and not in words or ways we are accustomed to. This is more challenging because many of us have not been taught the tremendous benefits of this space, which perhaps have not allowed us to pursue it with tenaciousness. Try it for thirty days, ten minutes twice a day. Don't allow frustration to cause you to quit. More is happening in you that you can't feel or see or detect with the senses. You will, however, begin to experience the benefits in many ways over time. Some of the benefits I have experienced are clearer thoughts, dreams, and visions, just to name a few. Power to overcome the old you is given to you in that space. Power to eat healthier is in that stillness space. Stillness is packed with hidden treasures that most will never receive because of the challenges that come to prevent you from getting in this space. Don't accept the thoughts that will come to trick you by telling you it's not working. Persevere the more by changing the ten minutes to fifteen, twenty, and thirty minutes consistently. This is going to be our new lifestyle, so be patient and take one step at a time. Enjoy the journey to wholeness.

Reflect

_____

_____

_____

_____

_____

_____

_____

_____

_____

_____

_____

_____

CHAPTER 15

Take Action

My journey started aggressively because I wanted to rid my body of pain. However, if you are not dealing with pain, sickness, or disease, but know that a change is needed, you can start slow and gradually take away things and add things. I was diagnosed with an infirmity, and I was in pain, so I took all starches and sugar out of my diet. I got relief from the pain within months, and the bonus was tremendous weight loss without trying. Forget focusing on weight loss. It's not real, and it will disappear like it was never there. Exercise was a part of my routine, but I never lost weight. However, I gained weight because they say muscle weighs more than fat. I was turning the fat into muscle, which did not result in weight loss but weight gain.

If you have been diagnosed by the world medical system with an infirmity, I recommend you remove starches and sugars out of your diet first. When you reach the threshold, which is different for each person, you will not miss the starches or sugars. I know you don't think that's possible, but I am a witness your body will not crave the starches or sugars. Fruit is very sweet to my palate now and satisfies the sugar taste whenever I think I want it.

Making the decision to begin this journey to wholeness is your first step. Choosing a heathier lifestyle is one of the greatest choices you will ever make. One of my greatest challenges when I began was finding things I could eat that were healthier choices. I compiled a list of items that I creatively put together throughout the time I have been on this journey that will help make your journey easier. You can build from my list and find other groups that are also on healthier lifestyles that share their recipes and then create some of your own and share with others who want to begin this lifestyle but don't know where or how to.

I found in talking to people who are interested in changing their lifestyle is that they are concerned with the cost. I live on a budget like many of you, but I know how important my health is, so I try to buy the best for the best (me) at the least cost possible. I go to the farmer's markets weekly. I have found fresh is best, and I buy organic as much as possible. Although there is lots of controversy surrounding organic fruits and vegetables, I try to choose organic fruits and veggies. I try to eat and juice as many green foods as possible because this is where the best nutrients are that will nourish my cells. I use all the different types of kale that I can find. I love the darker green kale for juicing. I started for months consuming smoothies daily, and then I started incorporating juicing mainly because of personal preference. One is cold, and one you can drink room temperature. Juicing is more concentrated, with mainly green veggies and some apples for sweeteners. Some people add fresh limes to give the bittersweet combo. I use spelt, chickpea, or kamut (any grain flour) to make a variety of what I call breakfast fritters. I got creative, which I have included throughout this book. I allowed my body to tell me what it wanted throughout the day. Try putting together various combinations of apple and banana, strawberry, blueberry, and banana, banana only, apple and blueberry, etc. I did that for months, and then I changed it up. Variety is the spice of life is my motto. I get bored with the same things every day as I am sure many of you do also. It is not the amount (portions) you eat that is important. It is more what you eat and how well it nourishes your cells. Breakfast changes often. If you are in a hurry, make just a couple pieces of spelt toast with organic vegan butter with no soy, and add flavored hummus as a topping. I juice a minimum of once a week (every day is my goal), and I try to make a smoothie twice a week. (You can be creative.) When I started this journey, it was challenging to find things that were healthy for me to eat. However, giving up was not an option. I kept searching and experimenting with what I learned is good for my body. I loved breakfast, so this was my greatest challenge to find healthy alternatives. My focus was finding breakfast foods that were healthy, and trust me, it was not easy. I found that as my taste buds changed, I could eat anything or not eat anything, because my body was no longer craving for those addictions. My focus is to give you a kick start so you don't give up and revert to the old habits. It is not easy, and if you fall back into the old habits, don't stay there. Get back up and start again.

Reflect

_____

_____

_____

_____

_____

_____

_____

_____

_____

_____

_____

_____

_____

CHAPTER 16

Modification

I love variety, so whatever comes to me is what I eat daily. I try to not eat anything on some days because I am in control of this body now. It no longer dictates to me through all the addictive foods I consumed. Fasting is excellent for us naturally and spiritually. It's normally not something anyone wants to do. However, the benefits are far greater than our wants. There are days I just drink water, which is vital for our bodies. We learned earlier that our bodies are 70 percent water. Detox is another place that gives our body a boost or revitalization. Do some studies on the benefits both naturally and spiritually. I want you to be free to follow your heart/spirit. I have found this works best for me. It is very important to drink as close to a gallon of spring water as you can. This is challenging for most, including me. What has worked best for me is first thing in the morning, it is good to drink at least sixteen ounces before eating or drinking anything else. I turn it up and don't stop until it's half gone, and I turn it up again and it's all gone. One bottle down and six more left to make the gallon. Seven sixteen-ounce (16.9) bottles will give you a gallon. Initially, if you are not a water drinker, you will visit the restroom quite often, but it will taper off as the body adjusts. This is quite an amazing machine that has been entrusted to us. Drinking water will help with the hunger feelings if you are a breakfast person. I also have found not drinking any liquids for one or two hours after eating solid foods helps your body digest the food. I have tried it, and it really works well for me. It was not easy at first, but amazingly, your body conforms to what is good. What I have not eliminated fully from my lifestyle is meat. However, I only eat it once a day. My goal is to not consume blood, starch, or processed sugars. It's a process; I like to say a journey. I skip days eating meats, and my body adjusts well. If I eat meat, it is no later than 4:00 p.m. Everyone has to choose how they start the journey. I would suggest you make choices according to your body and ailments. It is important to find what your body is deficient in and find the foods that have a high content of your deficiency and incorporate in your diet daily. A great example is many women over the age of fifty may find themselves calcium deficient or vitamin D deficient. My studies have found fresh dill, sea moss, papaya, bell pepper (I love the red ones), just to name a few, are all high in calcium. Also, dandelion is high in so many minerals the body needs. It has a very bitter taste, but I try to add it when I can. (What tastes good is not always good for us; keep that in mind.) I don't consume any meats such as pork, seafood, fish, or beef. I occasionally eat wild salmon. My lifestyle at this time consists of chicken and turkey in small amounts. You can get the protein from other things if you believe you need proteins that they say meat offers. (I am not convinced you can get anything healthy from something dead and processed.) I find that I don't have the feeling of hunger, so there are days I may eat very little, but my energy level is very good. I know now it is not important how much you eat, but what you eat is of utmost importance. Good food fuels the body, and it sustains you for longer periods of time than when you are consuming starches and sugars. My studies show sugar craves sugar and starches turn into sugar. Many of our diets are loaded with sugars, which form mucus and inflammation in our body, which compromises our cells and allows sickness and disease to enter our temples. When I want something sweet to drink, I will occasionally make limeade (key limes), and I sweeten it with maple grade B, agave syrup, or date sugar, which are delicious and fulfill that sweet tooth. The fritters are sweetened with grade B maple syrup, date sugar, or agave syrup in the batter only. I don't use syrup after they are made. I make spelt pancakes that my grands love and have included the recipe. I do not eat fried foods unless I fry it. I fry chicken/turkey strips in a small amount of grapeseed oil to satisfy my crunch desire. I have researched and found grapeseed, coconut oil, and avocado oil have high heating elements and are best for frying. Do not use olive oil for frying. However, you can add it to any of your food for taste after it is cooked because it does not have a high heating point.

Stop committing to diets. Instead, commit to a heathier lifestyle—a way of life different from the one you currently have. My studies show 80 percent of weight gain is what you eat. Remember, you are making this decision because you want to live a heathier life, you want to feel better, you want to live a long, healthy life, and you want your family and friends to choose a healthier lifestyle. Our children and grands need to learn a new healthier lifestyle, which can only come to them if we change. Most if not all diseases are not passed to us genetically. It is the way of eating that is passed to us generation after generation. I am committed to pass down a healthy lifestyle to my grands and great-grands. They will have choice and know the differences between good, healthy food and bad, unhealthy foods that cause sickness and diseases.

Reflect

Electric U

CHAPTER 17

Transition

Your health has no price tag. If you like the best things in life, then this is your chance to give your body the best. You are the most important person living (there is a treasure in earthen vessels, 2 Cor. 4:7). Your body houses that treasure.

An easy starting point to help you transition to an alkaline plant-based lifestyle is every day to commit to eating one thing healthy/alkaline/plant-based and removing one thing unhealthy. An alkaline diet/plant-based diet will nourish your cells and remove the taste of the unhealthy foods over time. The more you incorporate them in your daily regimen, the more you will notice your taste buds changing. It's a journey. We have eaten unhealthy for most of our lives, so it will take time to change. Be patient, and don't give up. There is a threshold, and you will make it. This is a guide that can help make this transition a little easier to get started.

Example

Breakfast—remove one of these items daily or weekly grits/eggs/sausage/bacon/cereals replace with

- ancient grains like amaranth, quinoa, teff, fonio (There are lots of free breakfast recipes on Google.)
- Spelt/rye breaded toasted instead of whole wheat, white bread.
- Coconut yogurt
- Spelt/pancakes/fritters
- Fruits/smoothies/juices with greens of your choice.

The goal is to add as many greens as possible to your daily intake. Greens have the highest nutrients that feed our cells. It's time to wake those cells up to help them to function the way God created them to function. You will think clearer thoughts. Your memory will improve. Your overall health will improve drastically, and you will feel good.

Reminder: Iron is one of the most important minerals our body needs. Add plant-based iron to your daily regimen. You can also use herbs that are high in iron and foods that are high in iron. Iron is to your blood as calcium is to your bone. Utilize Google to find what you need. A few examples are sarsaparilla, which has the highest concentration of iron, yellow dock root, elderberry, bugleweed, blue vervain, and burdock. They are all excellent iron sources.

Lunch—remove one daily or weekly pizza/hamburgers/ Chinese rice/fried food, etc. Replace with the following:

- Sandwich—rye or spelt bread, hummus, or avocado turkey/chicken (optional) with vegan mayonnaise.
- Wild rice is a healthy substitute for white rice for all the rice lovers.
- Incorporate, as often as possible, green salads/ green veggies of choice.
- If you don't eliminate meat right away, choose a meat of choice, baked or grilled only.
- Add walnuts/Brazilian nuts/currants for a fulfilling snack (homemade trail mix)
- If you love fried crunchy food, like I do, treat yourself weekly, but fry it yourself using spelt or chickpea flour and grapeseed or coconut oil.

Try to eat your heaviest meal at lunch or early afternoon. Smoothies will give you the full feeling most are used to.

Desserts: Replace cakes, cookies, candy, and ice cream with homemade desserts.

- blend strawberries, blueberries, mangos, etc., with coconut milk and freeze (Google recipes)
- fruit smoothies with any greens of choice/coconut milk or spring water
- coconut yogurt and add fresh fruit of choice.
- Make your own cookies. Just change the ingredients to healthier ingredients in your favorite recipe.

Dinner: Remove fried meats and rice. Replace with:

- green salads
- green veggies of choice (raw/bake/steam)
- try my vegan electrical chayote squash recipes

Key: As you transition to a healthy lifestyle, remember everything in moderation.

Look in the back of the book, and use some of the recipes to help you as you start your journey. I have been pretty creative. Thank You, Lord! The creative gift in me has been awakened. You will find He will awaken your creativeness also!

Reflect

_____

_____

_____

_____

_____

_____

_____

_____

_____

_____

_____

_____

_____

_____

CHAPTER 18

My hope and prayer is this book has been a tool that has awakened your spirit man to take charge of your body and soul so that your spirit man will lead you to a long and healthy life, which is what God created from the beginning of time for us all. I hope it will serve as a tool to help you get started on a healthier lifestyle. The threshold awaits you! Once you make it across, you will be well on your way to living the best life possible, having it *all*—all God promised and life more abundantly.

Let's see how much you have retained. Look at the recipe below. Cross out the unhealthy ingredients, and write a healthier choice to replace it. I will post my choices on the last page.

Original pancakes recipe includes the ingredients listed below. Create a healthier version by writing healthier ingredients next to the ones listed below. I have placed my choices on the last page of book.

Homemade Fruit Fritters or Pancakes

White flour
Eggs

Whole milk
Baking powder
White sugar
Butter
Canola oil

You can take any recipe you have and replace the unhealthy ingredients with healthier ingredients, and it will taste good!

These are helpful tools below that I have used and found to be helpful. I am sure they will assist you along your journey. More and more people are coming on board and are sharing helpful tools to make this transition a smoother one.

Dr. Sebi's Nutritional Guide is an excellent source to learn some of the foods that are alkaline

Chef Ahki is a great source for good recipes.
Ty's Conscious Kitchen is a source for recipes.
www.the figtreeonline.com (vitamins/herbs)
www.berlinnaturalbakery.com
www.nextgenerationherbalproducts.com
www.vitacost.com (foods/vitamins)

Created by Ms. C

All-Natural Healthier Choice Recipe Options:

Organic fresh or frozen fruits, ½ cup strawberries and/ or blueberries, and/or apple and/or (1–2) burro banana, blended with ¼ cup of almond or coconut milk or spring water. Add walnuts (optional). I add lots of walnuts because I love crunchy things, about a ½ cup. Mix with ¼ cup spelt flower and/or chickpea flour. Add 3–5 tbsp. of grade B maple syrup or raw blue or volcano agave (for added health benefits, add flaxseed or sea moss), use 1–2 tbsp. of coconut oil or grapeseed oil to coat the pan, and scoop ¼ cup or more of mixture into the pan and let it brown on each side.

Measurements vary depending upon how much you want to make. It should have the consistency of a pancake batter or a little thicker.

This is a nice breakfast treat to go along with your smoothie or fresh-made green juice. I have this at least once a week. They are a delicious electrical treat in place of traditional pancakes.

Do I have any creative innovators? Make up your own recipe using the above ingredients or other healthy ingredients.

Chayote/Zucchini Squash Spelt Noodles, Substitute Squash with Spinach/Callaloo

2 peeled and diced chayote squash (watch video of how to peel)
2–3 zucchini squash (dice in bite-size chunks)
1 chopped red bell pepper (your choice)
½ cup sliced portabella mushrooms (optional)
2–3 cups of spelt/kamut spiral noodle (season to taste, boil, and set aside)

Directions

Season as desired and cut into bite-size chunks. I cook it separately until it's the desired texture. I mix all ingredients together for a fabulous vegan one-pot dish.

Bake seasoned squash for 20 minutes (until tender) and zucchini for 10–15 minutes (until desired texture). I prefer it crunchy.

Zucchini Asparagus

1 zucchini squash diced
Slice of red bell pepper
1/2 cup of diced mushrooms
6 asparagus

Directions

Sauté asparagus in a tbsp grapeseed oil. Bake other ingredients in oven for 10 min. Season to taste.

Spiral Noodle with Chayote Squash

1 cup Kamut spiral noodles
5 cherry tomato (blanched)
1 chayote squash diced
2 cups callaloo
1 fried burro plantain
2 tbsp. grapeseed oil

Boil tomatoes until tender and mash. Boil kamut spiral 10–15 min, add tomatoes. Boil squash 10 min. Stir fry callaloo and add the squash.

As a healthy snack

Cut up cherry tomatoes
Cut up/dice cucumber
Sprinkle fresh dill (optional)
Sprinkle pink salt

Pepper (optional)

This is a great snack in between meals. It satisfies the crunch and is healthy

Squash Potluck

1–2 chayote squash diced
3–5 cherry tomatoes blanched
1–2 zucchini
1/4 c. red onions minced
1/4 fresh dill
1 stalk of green scallions
1/2 cup of seasoned spring water
1/2 tbsp. grapeseed oil

Season the squashes with favorite seasonings or just sprinkle with pink salt and pepper. Sauté all onions in oil for a few minutes, then add tomatoes and chayote squash and let simmer until tender. Add zucchini last if you like crunchy and let simmer for 3–5 minutes.

Hummus Wrap

1 romaine leaf of lettuce
2–3 scoops of lemon hummus
Toppings—chopped walnuts
Side of fried sweet plantains

Squash Dish

2 chayote squash diced
5 cherry tomatoes (blanched)
2 sliced Portobello mushrooms
Red onions
Bell pepper
Salt and pepper
Fresh dill to taste

Sauté onions and bell peppers in grapeseed oil. Add other ingredients. Add salt and pepper. Let simmer in its own juices slowly.

Butternut Sweet Potato

1 Butternut squash. Bake 30–45 min. until tender. Let cool and scoop seeds out, and then scoop out flesh and mash and add pure maple syrup or raw agave to taste, 1–2 tsp.

It tastes like sweet potatoes.

Banana Nut Muffins
(or substitute banana with apples or any desired fruit)

1 1/2 cups chopped walnuts (optional)
4 tbsp. grapeseed or coconut oil
2 tbsp. almond/walnut/vegan no soy butter, melted (optional)
1 tsp. pure organic vanilla bean (optional)
1/2 cup agave/maple syrup (to taste)

1/2 cup coconut yogurt
5 very ripe small/burro bananas, mashed
1 1/2 cups spelt/chickpea flour
½ tbs sea moss/Perrier water
1/2 tsp. pink Himalaya salt

Preheat oven to 350°F. Line muffin cups with paper liners. In a mixing bowl, whisk together oil, butter, vanilla, brown sugar, and yogurt.

Mash the banana, and stir into the mixture. Add chopped nuts. Stir in flour, Perrier water, and sea salt. To avoid tough and dry muffins, do not overmix batter. Fill muffins cups 2/3 full or about 1/2 cup of batter. Bake in preheated oven for 23 to 25 minutes, or until muffin tops are golden brown. Be careful to avoid baking muffins too long or they will be dry.

Ms C healthier changes to the recipe quiz are:

Spelt flour and chickpea flour
No eggs
Coconut or almond milk
Sea moss/Perrier water
Maple syrup/date sugar/agave syrup
Grapeseed oil/coconut oil

Printed in the United States
By Bookmasters